Sudden Death in Childhood

This book is dedicated to the memory of children who have died suddenly and unexpectedly

Commissioning Editor: Susan Young
Development Editor: Catherine Jackson
Project Manager: Samantha Ross
Designer: George Ajayi
Illustrations Manager: Bruce Hogarth

Sudden Death in Childhood: Support for the Bereaved Family

Ann Dent SRN PhD (Social Policy)
Honorary Research Fellow in Child Health, Bristol University, UK

Alison Stewart RGN RM RHV PhD (Nsg)
Senior Lecturer & Postgraduate Programme Leader, School of Nursing,
Otago Polytechnic, New Zealand

Forewords by

Gordon Riches BEd MA (Ed) MA
Head of Sociology, University of Derby, UK

Jean Simons BA (Hons) MSc CQSW
Assistant Director, Family Policy, Great Ormond Street Hospital and Joint
Co-ordinator, Child Death Helpline, UK

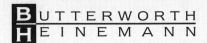
BUTTERWORTH
HEINEMANN

EDINBURGH LONDON NEW YORK OXFORD PHILADELPHIA ST LOUIS SYDNEY TORONTO 2004

BUTTERWORTH-HEINEMANN
An imprint of Elsevier Limited

First published 2004

ISBN 0 7506 5646 8

British Library Cataloguing in Publication Data
A catalogue record for this book is available from the British Library

Library of Congress Cataloging in Publication Data
A catalog record for this book is available from the Library of Congress

Notice
Medical knowledge is constantly changing. Standard safety precautions must be followed, but as new research and clinical experience broaden our knowledge, changes in treatment and drug therapy may become necessary or appropriate. Readers are advised to check the most current product information provided by the manufacturer of each drug to be administered to verify the recommended dose, the method and duration of administration, and contraindications. It is the responsibility of the practitioner, relying on experience and knowledge of the patient, to determine dosages and the best treatment for each individual patient. Neither the Publisher nor the authors assume any liability for any injury and/or damage to persons or property arising from this publication.

The Publisher

Disclaimer
The central thesis of this book is the complexity and diversity of grief. Hence definitive statements about practice cannot be made. Each health professional has to use their professional judgement when making assessments and planning care. The considerations for practice proposed in this book are exactly that; they offer ideas for health professionals to consider. Therefore, the authors and publisher take no responsibility for readers' interpretations and any subsequent actions. Decisions in practice are the responsibility of the health professional who holds current registration of competency to practice. While every effort has been made to ensure that information is accurate at the time of going to press, it remains the responsibility of each health professional to ensure that their practice is consistent with current research, relevant legislation and the policies of employers.

The URLs quoted were correct at the time of going to press, however, information on the Internet, including URLs, is subject to constant change.

 ELSEVIER SCIENCE your source for books, journals and multimedia in the health sciences

www.elsevierhealth.com

The publisher's policy is to use **paper manufactured from sustainable forests**

Printed in China

Contents

APPENDICES 199

Forewords

Things happen that cannot be put into words. Some experiences are beyond the capacity of the mind to comprehend or the emotions to contain. Sudden, traumatic unexpected deaths of children are beyond description. Healthcare workers, researchers, psychologists and counsellors have, for years, struggled to find words that capture the devastation that accompanies miscarriage, still birth, sudden infant death, and deaths in childhood and young adulthood. Theories of attachment, loss and grief come and go. We have never had so many models for making sense of what happens when intimate relationships are conceived, realised, taken-for-granted and then are arbitrarily, apparently wantonly, destroyed. The ties binding mother to father, surviving children to their parents, families to grandparents and the wider family to a myriad of friendship and public networks are strained, often to breaking point.

Thankfully, the clinical model of grief (if it ever existed in pure form) is retreating. Psychology of individual attachment and loss no longer monopolises the range of conceptual tools that we use to explore bereavement. Most importantly, the dead themselves are increasingly recognised as exerting a continuing influence on the living – something they have always done in other cultures. Of the many forces that have helped shape contemporary theories of bereavement – sometimes referred to as 'new models' of grief – the role of bereavement support groups has to be acknowledged. It is a salutary but uplifting experience to work with groups such as TCF (The Compassionate Friends), SANDS (Still-birth and Neo-natal Death Society), SAMM (Support After Murder and Manslaughter), and SOBS (Survivors of Bereavement through Suicide). They, along with many others noted in Appendix 1, have diverted our attention from clinical settings to support networks. Grief as 'pathology' has now given way to a post-modern appreciation of the diverse and idiosyncratic ways in which individuals, relationships and families survive sudden and traumatic losses. These 'self-help' groups have aided researchers in identifying the importance of informal social networks and the value of shared sub-cultures of loss in aiding the resilience of long-term survivors.

A group of bereaved parents from one such support group, including some who are practising nurses and midwives of many years' experience, offered the following suggestions when I asked for their advice in writing this foreword:

*Remind them (health care workers) that, 'There, but for the grace of God, go they ...' They may be trained professionals, with lots of experience of death. But that will mean nothing when it happens to their child. Remind them that it takes **years** to learn to live a normal life again. Remind them that this isn't ordinary normal. It is a totally new kind of 'normal'. We never go back to being the same people we once were.*

Remind them of the pressure everyone puts on us to get better, to get over it – some of that pressure coming directly from them. Remember that bereavement is not a medical condition and grief is not an illness that can be cured. Remind them that, unless they have been through it, they cannot begin to imagine how fundamentally and irrevocably their lives will be changed. I pray that they will never find out, but they need to be aware that it could happen to them as easily as it has to us.

Tell them that nothing can replace open, unconditional compassion and a willingness to be there, through everything, for the long haul. Tell them how lonely, disoriented, devastated and isolated we feel and how hurtful well-meaning cliches can be: 'You need to move on. … Focus on having another', 'Time is a greater healer even though you cannot see it at the moment'. Remind them that the death of my child is not the same as the death of their parent or their partner.

Tell them that we appreciate them and that often they are marvellous. Many of us could not have survived without them, and we genuinely appreciate their work, even though sometimes we have funny ways of showing it. (One bereaved mother gave an example of a GP who used to arrange double appointments. 'She would have a box of tissues ready and would say, when I was sobbing, "Don't rush. … Take your time." ')

Tell them what we most need is an opportunity to share our children's lives so that it does not seem weird or morbid to talk about the dead. Tell them that we, or our partners, or our children might need help and time to feel brave enough and comfortable enough to talk. Tell them that the biggest problem is that no one really has the time to listen. Few want to listen – especially later when we start to find words to talk about it. Tell them, if they haven't got time, to pass on the contact details of bereavement support groups because these national help-lines will provide the names of people who do, at least in part, understand what we are going through.

It is a privilege to be invited to write the foreword to this exceptional book that so beautifully demonstrates a genuine respect for the feelings and voices of bereaved people. Ann and Alison have produced an invaluable resource for those who offer support during and after the sudden death of a child. Their writing reflects the work of two very experienced and sensitive practitioners. They have, in these pages, constructed a bridge between the professional culture of health workers and the all too hidden culture of bereaved families. In doing so, they have connected theory with practice, individual psychology with the social context upon which it rests, and intensely private reactions with the culture of beliefs and assumptions that inform all our thoughts and emotional responses. Not only does this book introduce us to current debates and issues within bereavement research it also makes them highly relevant through the carefully chosen case examples of people who have experienced sudden bereavement.

Although ostensibly aimed at nurses and midwives, this accessible text is of value to anyone working within health or counselling services. Its potential readership is large. Teachers, social and community workers, bereavement self-help and support groups, and individuals touched by their own losses, will discover insight, practical advice and personal reassurance from this carefully researched and thoughtfully presented book.

Gordon Riches, 2004

The authors of this meticulously researched, logically presented and beautifully clear book promote the practice of 'family awareness' rather than the more usually heard phrase 'working with families', and this sets the tone for truly family-focussed care. 'Family awareness' entails exploring and understanding the meaning of the child's death for each of the people in the child's important circle, whether they are grandparents, siblings, friends, child minders or others. Recognising and acknowledging the needs and feelings of these family members, rather than imposing a professionally led agenda for bereavement support, is the focus of all work. This approach respects the particular family's experience of grief and enables them to describe their own individual needs; it acknowledges 'normality' in relation to individual resilience and diversity, rather than requiring assessment against a professionally pre-ascribed concept.

In order to explore, establish and understand the meaning for these individual family members, the healthcare professional primarily needs appropriate listening skills, rather than training in 'bereavement counselling'. The authors acknowledge that the task of really listening to grieving people is not easy, and it is the skill with which many healthcare professionals are least comfortable. They are more used to giving information to establish their expertise; reassuring rather than acknowledging uncertainty; doing, rather than 'merely being alongside'. Any bereaved parent knows and probably accepts that not even the most experienced professional can truly 'understand' or 'make it better', but will usually acknowledge that the person who was most helpful to them was the one who 'could listen'. The emergence and establishment of parent-to-parent self help, befriending and support organisations is testament to the altruism and determination of very many bereaved parents to provide, usually in a voluntary capacity, the 'just listening' to others in their own circumstances.

A bereaved parent will usually be able to listen to and acknowledge what another bereaved parent has to say about their feelings or their experiences. However, a volunteer from the Child Death Helpline said that from her own experience, and that of many of her colleagues, she had concluded that, 'other people, including many professionals, are simply scared of bereaved parents'. A health visitor, quoted by the authors, gave her opinion that supporting bereaved parents is a job for which many in her profession are 'hugely ill-prepared and consequently dread'. This professional fear sadly adds to the isolation that bereaved parents feel when a friend does not call, or an acquaintance crosses the road in embarrassment and confusion. Many professionals are similarly reluctant to approach a bereaved parent without 'extra training'.

The authors rightly emphasise the need for healthcare professionals in contact with suddenly bereaved families to be aware of the particular issues and sensitivities of all the family members involved. They use the term, 'considerations for practice' in keeping with the non-prescriptive tone. They do not assume, perhaps seemingly against current recommendations, that a bereaved person cannot be appropriately supported without the professional having special qualifications. On this point, the development of bereavement advisor posts in paediatric trusts is to be applauded if the resultant awareness-raising benefits all healthcare professionals' confidence and thus the effectiveness of their contact with bereaved families. However, if 'bereavement work' comes to be seen as the province of only specialised professionals this may deskill the nurse, midwife, or health visitor who needs to be able to offer immediate support.

Although the sudden death of a child is the most shocking and devastating event anyone must face, the authors believe, and evidence, that the skills the healthcare professionals are trained to use in communication through all stages of the patient journey, are the appropriate skills required to support a suddenly bereaved family.

Particular situations, which may benefit from referral to a specialist service are outlined, and the main contemporary and influential theories of grief and mourning are helpfully summarised and reviewed. However, the intention is not to overspecialize support work with bereaved families, but to emphasise the essential normality of even the most unexpected reaction, which a suddenly bereaved parent or grieving family member may experience, and about which they will most likely need sympathetic discussion and reassurance rather than specialist referral.

Although this text book is aimed specifically at nurses, midwives and health visitors, the concepts discussed and the skills promoted are entirely relevant for any professional involved with the care of all families who have suffered the death of a child, of any age, in any circumstance.

It is a privilege to have been asked to provide a brief foreword to this book and a pleasure to commend it to the list of 'classics' in the field of bereavement care and support, providing a model of good practice for all health care professionals.

Jean Simons, 2004

Preface

Bev Gatenby, whose daughter died suddenly, chose as the title of her book *For the rest of our lives – after the death of a child*. It is a reminder that the family world changes forever when a child dies. In such a situation, what care can nurses and midwives offer?

Current practice for bereavement care is informed by interpretations of writings about grief derived from clinical practice and research. The last 15 years have seen new ways to conceptualise grief, with an emphasis on the cognitive processes by which people seek to make their own individual meaning of the experience. This represents a shift away from more universal theories of grief to focus on the diversity of ways in which people live with their loss and develop different forms of relationship with the deceased. In addition, there is an increasing awareness of the contexts in which individuals are bereaved. Individuals do not grieve in isolation. The beliefs, values and expectations of others, such as family and friends, can shape individuals' experience of bereavement.

So, how do nurses and midwives make decisions about care for bereaved family members? This book focuses on the sudden death of babies and children during pregnancy or childhood. It is the resource for which health professionals have asked since our first book *At a loss – bereavement care when a baby dies* became out of print. It is based on our joint clinical experiences as nurse, midwife and health visitor working with bereaved family members, integrated with the research we have undertaken and a range of writings about bereavement. Throughout the book, we explore contexts and perspectives of grief with stories and comments from bereaved family members. We do not provide definitive statements for practice but identify some considerations for practice. These require adaptation by each health professional to suit the situation and family members with whom they are working.

Ann Dent
Alison Stewart
UK and New Zealand 2004

Acknowledgements

We would like to thank all the bereaved families and health professionals who have shared their experiences and ideas with us over the years. They have taught us to appreciate the diversity of grief and the complexities of clinical practice. They have helped to make this book possible. We thank all the parents and grandparents who participated in the research that we undertook and who have consented to the inclusion of their comments in this book. In particular, Rose wrote a story with the assistance of John, which has been included in Chapter 3. Jenny and Rochelle, Matthew's sister, have given permission for their work, which was presented in Alison's doctoral thesis and which is due for publication during 2003 with Nursing Praxis International, to be included in this text. In recognition of the support that parents, grandparents and siblings have given to our research and this book, some of the royalties from the text are donated to a UK group for bereaved families. We are also grateful to all at Elsevier for their support and help in producing this book, and to Gill Gill and Toity Deave for their comments.

Ann pays special tribute to Richard, her husband, who has shown much tolerance and patience over the years to allow her to continue with her work. She would also like to thank all in the Department of Child Health, especially Professor Peter Fleming, who guided her into this work, and to Peter Blair for his patient and willing help on statistics and methodology. She is also grateful to all in her support group who have encouraged and supported her over the years, and to her family and friends who have been constant companions and supported her in many ways.

Alison acknowledges the support she has had from John, Phil, Judy and members of the Baby Bereavement Group. She has appreciated the encouragement of colleagues at Otago Polytechnic and the University of Otago, in particular, Shona Neehoff, Barbara Lowen, Alison Dixon, Rhondda Davies, Kate Pledger and Barry Taylor. She also appreciates the commitment of research participants who have been constant in their desire to see the stories of grandparent bereavement made available to health professionals.

About the authors

ANN DENT

As one of the first Macmillan community nurses Ann helped to set up and run St Peter's Hospice in Bristol. Subsequently she worked to achieve community care for dying children and their families in the South West region. As a Macmillan nurse consultant she was involved in setting up services nationally for children with cancer and running many workshops for professionals on care of the dying child and the family. She was one of three nurses to set up the first hospice in Russia.

More recently she has conducted research into support for families after sudden child death at the Department of Child Health in Bristol University, giving papers nationally and internationally on her work. She initiated and was involved in running two International Conferences on *Children & Death* in the UK.

Over the years she has helped to set up and run two branches of Cruse (a voluntary bereavement agency). For 4 years she was chair of the consultant panel of the *Child Bereavement Network* and is currently chair of the *Bereavement Research Forum*.

ALISON STEWART

Alison has been involved in clinical practice, research and education relating to bereavement following the death of a child during pregnancy or childhood. This has included working with individual members of families, family groups and members of mutual help groups. Following her work as Avon Infant Mortality Coordinator, she co-authored a book with Ann entitled *At a loss* (Stewart & Dent 1994).

Over the years Alison has been involved with research studies, supporting local mutual help groups and developing information materials and workshops for both bereaved families and those who work with them, such as health professionals and teachers. Recently her role has included developing and teaching a postgraduate paper in a Master of Nursing which focuses on transition, bereavement and change within nursing practice. She has had a particular interest in the experiences of bereaved grandparents and in 2000 completed her doctorate in nursing, which explores perspectives of grandparents' grief through the stories of grandparents and parents.

REFERENCES

Stewart A, Dent A 1994 At a Loss. Baillière Tindall, Edinburgh, UK

Setting the scene

The sudden death of a child holds different meanings for different members of bereaved families. This is illustrated by the comments from Donald and Jenny.

Donald reflected on his view of grief after the deaths of his brother, father and daughter Gracie.

> *I think, for everybody, coming to terms with it is the big one. I mean grief for everybody is different but it is being able to talk about it afterwards. We, as a family, are getting better at grief. There are aspects of every family death that are different. Like, whether you know they are going to die and how long you have got to come to terms with it, the age differences between the kids and the parents or brothers.*

Jenny shared her thoughts several years after her grandson's death.

> *I had never thought before about the possibility that my grandchild might die. Jordan's death has made me more aware of how tenuous life is – to get pregnant and have a baby 9 months later seemed normal and easy. But I now know how often pregnancies do go wrong. So, our faith in the future isn't automatic – we still have hope but it is always tempered with caution and the realisation that life can, and does, go badly wrong.*

Comments and stories such as those from Donald and Jenny form the heart of this book, which is about the experiences that parents, siblings and grandparents may face when a child dies suddenly. For many family members, the world turns upside down after the death of a child; people face living in a changed world. Health professionals, watching distressed family members, can feel powerless to remove their pain. How can nurses and midwives help to support bereaved families?

In this book we integrate experiences of family members with research findings and experience from working with bereaved families to develop **considerations** for nursing and midwifery practice. These ideas reflect the experiences of **some** family members and **some** ways of working with family members. We make no claim that these ideas will suit all individuals; instead they are considerations. This opening section sets the scene by reviewing:

- sudden death during pregnancy and childhood in England and Wales
- the context and beliefs that underpin this book
- an overview of the content in subsequent chapters.

SUDDEN DEATH DURING PREGNANCY AND CHILDHOOD

In many situations where a child dies, the death is sudden. It occurs quickly, unexpectedly and often without warning. Situations where there is no prewarning include a parent who finds their baby dead in their cot or children killed instantaneously in an accident or vehicle crash. In other situations, there may be moments, or even days, when treatment may seek to avert death: for example when life support is withdrawn from a child after an accident, a mother has several days of spot bleeding at 12 weeks of gestation then miscarries, or a baby, born unexpectedly at 24 weeks of gestation, dies a few days later in the neonatal intensive care unit (NICU). In these situations, the family are facing an unexpected situation for which they have had little warning. The commonality in these examples is that the family were generally anticipating that all was well with the child and then **suddenly** the situation changed and their child was dead. In a wide range of situations, we have listened to family members describe their child's death as 'sudden'; it is their interpretation of the experience. Such a perception is presented in Marie's description of her granddaughter's death.

> *It was sudden to us. I mean it was not like she had been ill for months or even weeks with cancer or something. She was fine during pregnancy, fine when born, she seemed OK, then a bit unwell and then she died. It was only days. There was no time to prepare or take it in. It just felt so sudden. That is what I still remember a year later – the **suddenness**.*

By framing this book about 'sudden death', we have been guided by the ways in which family members have described their experiences. We have used **sudden** to include both instantaneous deaths and situations where the death was unexpected but may have been preceded by several days of care, often designed to avert the death. Families may perceive both situations as sudden deaths in terms of the child having been generally healthy in previous days and months; then, the circumstances suddenly changed. Another element of such sudden deaths is, as Jenny described at the beginning of the chapter, the belief that children do not die and that pregnancies are normal and healthy. This can enhance the sense that the death was both sudden and unexpected because, as one grandmother explained, '*children are not expected to die in Western society*'. So, is sudden death during pregnancy or childhood rare?

Information from the Office for National Statistics for deaths in England and Wales during 2001 indicates that many babies and children died in circumstances that may have been sudden and/or unexpected for their families (Office for National Statistics 2002a,b).

- 3157 babies were stillborn
- 2108 babies aged less than 28 days died from causes such as pregnancy and labour-related events, congenital anomalies and conditions related to immaturity
- 195 infants aged from 28 days to 4 years died from sudden infant death syndrome (SIDS)
- 85 children aged from 28 days to 14 years died from meningococcal infection

- 287 children aged from 28 days to 14 years died as a result of accidents including causes related to traffic, poisons, water and electricity
- 82 adolescents aged from 10 to 19 years died from intentional self-harm.

These numbers do not include the extent of death during pregnancy, such as miscarriage or late fetal loss before 24 weeks of gestation. Even this brief summary illustrates that many families, and therefore health professionals, encounter the sudden death of a child in their lives. While official statistics reveal the number of deaths, they do not reflect the extent or nature of bereavement and grief that follows such deaths. The nature of such grief can be complex because it involves a child, a family and the death is sudden.

SUDDEN DEATH OF A CHILD IN THE FAMILY

For each child who dies several, sometimes many people are left bereaved. Like a stone dropped into water, one child's death creates a 'death ripple' (Jordan et al 1993, p. 425). This ripple of bereavement means that everyone in the family has been bereaved: parents, grandparents and siblings. The ripple also touches the extrafamilial setting including friends of an older child, colleagues of parents, neighbours, teachers, acquaintances in community groups and health professionals. In addition, the ripple of bereavement can extend forward over time, so that the experience will remain with an individual and may influence future decisions, behaviours and feelings.

Whether sudden or expected, the death of a child is generally perceived as untimely. It challenges the anticipated sequence of events in Western society where grandparents and parents expect to predecease their children. Death brings a primary loss – absence of the person. It also brings secondary losses, which alter existing roles, relationships and everyday activities within the family. As the comments from Donald and Jenny indicate, people often struggle to make sense of the changed world. Most importantly, an individual's bereavement does not exist in isolation. The experience of bereavement is shaped by the surrounding contexts, such as the family (Rosenblatt 2002). The support, comments, beliefs and expectations of family members, friends, local communities and wider society can affect the ways in which individuals cope with, and make sense of, their bereavement.

Writing from the context of deaths such as stroke, homicide and vehicle crash, Doka (1996) noted that grief after sudden death may be difficult and often intensified. Reasons include lack of opportunity to say farewell, the sudden change to the world as it was known by the survivor and having unanswered questions about the death. These occur in many situations where a baby or child dies suddenly. Many family members have questions about 'What happened?' and 'Why?' after deaths such as stillbirth, SIDS, drowning, accidents and natural disasters. The nature and circumstances of some sudden deaths can mean that family members' experiences of bereavement includes contact with a range of agencies – all of which can contribute to delays, uncertainty and even distress. For example, there may be involvement of the police and criminal justice system after homicide or vehicle crash. When the cause of sudden death is unknown, there may be involvement of the coroner and a postmortem may be required. In addition, the circumstances of some sudden deaths preclude the opportunity to 'say goodbye' to the dead child, possibly leaving regrets for surviving family members about what was said or unsaid. All these aspects of sudden death can contribute to the complexity of grief experienced by parents, grandparents, siblings, friends and others.

THE FOCUS OF THIS BOOK

In this book, we have explored some of the challenges that families face when a baby or child dies suddenly. We have not assumed that the experiences of all families are the same; the meaning of bereavement is unique to the individual. However, we believe that there are some issues that many parents face when a child dies suddenly, in a range of circumstances from pregnancy to adolescent years. These can offer broad considerations for nursing and midwifery practice with bereaved families. Some of the considerations may also be relevant to situations where death of a child is not sudden and may have been anticipated. We have not assumed that stillbirth is the beginning of childhood. For some families, miscarriage or ectopic pregnancy represents the death of their 'baby' and the ending of a relationship with their dreamed-of child. However, we do not claim that the experiences of parents whose baby miscarries is the same as those whose teenager is murdered; only that all parents are facing the sudden loss of their child. So, what are the ways in which health professionals can support families at this time?

Given some of the potential complexities of bereavement following the sudden death of a child, it is not surprising that many health professionals are unsure how to help bereaved families. Consequently, numerous books and articles have been written to support and inform clinical practice. This book is one of many such resources available to health professionals. It is not a definitive text; it offers possibilities and not prescriptions for practice. It includes material that is of relevance to both preregistration and postregistration study. However, it does not include the level of detailed debate that is present when an entire book is focused on a single issue. Such texts provide valuable further reading and we have listed these in references and reading resources. Neither does this text offer detailed management of physical care for women experiencing threatened miscarriage or attempted resuscitation of a child. Other texts offer this detail. Our focus has been on supporting bereaved family members. Therefore, this book offers a discussion of issues relevant to nursing and midwifery practice at the beginning of the 21st century. Our aims through the book have been to:

- include the experiences of some family members described in their own words
- discuss a range of published materials including the contexts that influence individuals' grief and the relationships that family members develop with a dead child
- consider ways in which health professionals can work confidently and sensitively with bereaved people.

The book has focused on issues that are relevant to nurses and midwives working in both hospital and community settings. In a hospital environment this includes midwives in a delivery unit or postnatal wards and nurses in gynaecology wards, neonatal/paediatric intensive care units or accident and emergency departments. From a primary health care perspective, the book has relevance for practice nurses, health visitors and midwives whose practice is based on community settings. To describe the wide range of roles where registered nurses, midwives or health visitors work with families, we have used the terms 'nurses and midwives' or 'health professionals'. We also note that relevant documents, legislation and statistics referred to in this text are generally applicable to England and Wales. Health professionals working in other areas need to be aware that there may be some differences and source appropriate information and legislation.

THE CONTEXT OF THE BOOK

Critical appraisal of both research and other sources of knowledge is fundamental to maintaining current, appropriate and professional practice. So, what is the knowledge base underpinning this book? In this section, we make explicit the beliefs that have shaped our interpretation of information about bereavement, grief and clinical practice.

OUR BELIEFS ABOUT THE WORLD

This is not a text written from an objective stance. We fully acknowledge that our beliefs shape how we view the world. In this book we have emphasised our beliefs that individuals make sense of the world, individuals do not grieve in isolation and each person has their own story. These beliefs have developed from reflection about our own personal experiences as members of families, from working with bereaved families and from offering education workshops for health professionals. We have integrated this experience with our interpretation of research studies and other writings. Consequently, this book represents our view of working with bereaved families. It is located in 2003 but our views will continue to change as we have new experiences and ideas.

CONSTRUCTIONS OF REALITY: MAKING SENSE OR MEANING

We believe that individuals actively interpret and make sense of situations, ideas and events to create a reality. This has been described in various writings including *The social construction of reality* by Berger and Luckmann (1966). For an overview see Nadeau (1998). The individual constructs a view of the world using existing beliefs, values, knowledge and previous experiences. This is reflected in the comment of Riches and Dawson (2000, p. 16) that *'bereaved people are active individuals, making choices as they deal with their experience of loss. Parents and siblings are not simply victims of circumstance.'* From this perspective, grief can be viewed as a transition from an *'assumptive world'*, which *'contains everything that we assume to be true on the basis of our previous experience'* (Parkes 1988, p. 56). A death requires individuals to reconstruct a view of a new assumptive world that incorporates the death. Previous experiences of loss and change, which are often gained as part of growing up in a family, can influence how individuals cope with bereavement and reconstruct their view of reality.

The key issue for this text is that there are potentially many constructions of reality. Individuals may have different constructions of the same situation or event. This is apparent in the stories and comments of family members in Chapters 3–5. For example, two grandparents may share the same event of experiencing the sudden death of their grandchild. Their **realities** of being bereaved may have some shared aspects such as 'concern for the parents' and also some unique aspects such as 'he was my only grandchild' or 'he was my sixth grandchild'. Just as constructions of reality may vary between individuals, the same individual can have different constructions at different points in time. For example, a parent cannot find a way to integrate their child's death into their assumptive world. The death may represent chaos and uncertainty when previously life had been familiar and known. Several months later, the parent might adopt a spiritual belief that there is life after death and find that this offers a way to live with, and make a meaning from, the death.

FAMILY AND CULTURE AS CONTEXTS TO GRIEF

Individuals gain their experiences, beliefs, values and ideas from roles and relationships that they hold in the social and cultural contexts within which they live. These influence the ways in which reality is constructed and can shape an individual's grief by offering support or constraints. The work of Walter (1999) and Riches and Dawson (2000) is discussed in Chapter 2. These offer valuable sociological perspectives for clinical practice. In particular, Riches and Dawson's (2000) work is of particular relevance to this book. The authors, a sociologist and bereavement coordinator, undertook sensitive research with over 50 bereaved parents and siblings in England during the mid-1990s. The deaths of the children, aged from unborn to 30 years, were predominantly 'sudden' and included accidents, stillbirths, cot death and voluntary termination. Riches and Dawson identified that personal, social and cultural resources are available to bereaved individuals and that these influence the ways in which people cope with their grief. The resources proposed by Riches and Dawson are described more fully on pp. 39–41. Figure 1.1 (p. 4) represents their idea that these resources are located within the contexts surrounding bereaved individuals.

The contexts and resources are interrelated. For example, the surrounding cultural context includes societal beliefs about grieving that may influence the social resources available to an individual. A friend who believes that grief is something that people should 'get over' may say to a bereaved mother 6 months after the death 'Are you still crying?' This may give a message to the bereaved mother that support is not available, that an opportunity to talk about her child does not exist and that she is expected to hide her bereavement and 'get on' with her life. Conversely, her mother, the child's grandmother, may believe in the value of listening to bereaved people. Her willingness to spend time with her daughter and to talk about the grandchild may offer the support that the daughter needs to cope with, and make sense of, her experience. In both instances, the beliefs and behaviours of the friend and grandmother will have been shaped by their surrounding context including societal beliefs, representations of grief in the media and personal experiences. In the wider cultural context, legislation may shape parents' experience of bereavement. For example, babies born dead before 24 weeks of gestation in England and Wales do not receive a birth or death certificate. Consequently, parents may feel that their babies have little social value, since there is no legislative acknowledgement of their loss and grief (Malacrida 1998). Hence the contexts surrounding individuals provide resources that influence their experiences of bereavement.

So how do individuals use resources from different contexts to make meaning of their experience? We believe that conversations and stories offer a way for some people. They also offer a way for health professionals to learn about others' experiences.

STORIES AND REFLECTION

People tell stories as part of everyday life. Stories can offer a way to describe the world in which people live and help to make sense of their experiences. For some people, stories are a means of reconstructing a view of the world after a change, such as death. This is not to assume that stories suit everyone, nor that stories have to exist in any particular form. Stories may be thoughts or conversations told to oneself, told to others or written in a journal. They may be memories and comments shared with family and friends who knew the deceased. Walter (1996) described, in the biographical model of grieving, that conversations with others who knew the deceased can help to build a story of self and the deceased. As Nadeau (1998) indicated, stories form ways for family members to make some meaning in a changed world. This is apparent in some of the quotations and stories that we have included in Chapters 3 and 5. Stories are also part of various therapeutic approaches to bereavement such as group/individual counselling sessions or working with a narrative therapist to share insights and gain new meanings (e.g. McCall 1989, White & Epston 1990, Neimeyer 2001a).

The perspective that stories offer a way to make meaning and learn about the world is of central importance to this text. Nurses and midwives are generally skilled listeners. Central to health-promoting practice is listening to the stories that other people tell as they describe, make sense of and live with their illness or health experience. Listening to stories is an important consideration for practice with bereaved families. In addition, the stories that family members tell offer health professionals the opportunity to gain insight into the experiences of those for whom they are caring. This, in turn, can inform practice and help professionals to care for bereaved family members. Therefore, we have included quotations and stories to illuminate the different ways that family members seek to make sense of their bereavement. As Leibrich (1999, p. 183) described, there is *'wisdom'* to be gained from stories: *'… information is just about facts – things that are usually told to us. Knowledge comes from integrating those facts. But wisdom comes through understanding – standing **under** knowledge and allowing the insight we gain from our own experience to illuminate knowledge. This is what is in these stories – wisdom.'* Our writing can offer ideas and considerations for practice, but it is the stories of people such as Rose (p. 48) and Jenny (p. 92) that will be remembered long after people have finished reading this book. From an educational perspective, stories offer a means to share ideas and learn about practice by exploring, and then expanding, issues through reflection. This requires using skills such as self-awareness, description of events and critical analysis (see McDrury & Alterio 2002). As reflective practice is an integral part of the competencies for registration as a nurse or midwife (UK Central Council for Nursing, Midwifery and Health Visiting 2001, 2000), it seems pertinent to emphasise the importance of stories as a means for reflection on practice. We return to this in Chapter 9.

EVIDENCE AND PRACTICE

During the 1990s, the expectation that evidence will underpin practice has emerged in government documents, clinical practice and competencies for registration. Using evidence in practice is related to managing health service delivery, maintaining clinical effectiveness and making decisions with clients about optimum choices for care. As Dawes (1999, p. ix) noted, evidence-based practice is underpinned by a philosophy of *'never taking for granted your own practice'.* Throughout this book we have emphasised the need to question and reflect on practice with bereaved families. Over the years, we have offered many workshops to enable health professionals to explore their practice with bereaved families. Sometimes we meet colleagues who want to *know* how to care for bereaved people; some want a checklist for practice. The debates we have during the workshops centre not on a checklist but on questions. Why is care being offered in this way? What are the assumptions that shape practice? How does professional judgement use research and assessment to plan bereavement care? What informs and shapes practice with bereaved people? We discuss some of these issues in subsequent chapters.

As we note in Chapter 6, the variety of interventions, bereavement events, sample sizes and outcome measures hampers attempts to compare one form of bereavement care with another. This can limit health professionals' ability to reach conclusions about 'how best' to care for bereaved people. Who decides what is 'best'? What is 'best' for one person may not be for another. Increasingly, there has been a *'de-emphasis on universal syndromes of grieving'* (Neimeyer 2001b, p. 3) and a recognition of the ways in which grief varies according to different relationships, circumstances of death and family settings. This means that we have proposed **considerations for practice**. We must stress that these are neither prescriptive nor a checklist. We make no claim that they apply to all bereaved people. They are considerations for practice that need to be adapted to each individual and situation. By keeping up to date with research, health professionals can adapt the considerations to suit their practice.

In this book, we have used various forms of information or 'evidence' to explore questions such as 'What informs current practice?' and 'How might we care for bereaved parents?' These include:

- a national and a randomised controlled trial of health visitor support to families after sudden child death
- listening to bereaved families over many years working in various roles and settings as nurse, midwife and health visitor
- listening to the perspectives of health professionals who attend our workshops
- a wide range of theoretical writings and research.

For the last, our literature searches have extended across journals and databases in the fields of nursing, allied health, midwifery, psychology, medicine and sociology. However, our writing inevitably reflects the bias of literature sourced primarily from the UK, USA, Australia and New Zealand. Similarly, we acknowledge that our own research informs the text, but we make no claim to generalise it to all parents or grandparents. In our research, the people who chose to participate were motivated to describe their experiences. The experiences of other people, who were unable to participate for whatever reason, do not have a voice in the book. Therefore, we are offering insights from the experiences of **some** people.

RESEARCH PERSPECTIVES

To appreciate the research from which some of our ideas for practice are derived we have provided a short overview of the methodology and findings. Both research studies were approved by relevant ethics committees. For further detail see Dent et al 1996, Dent (2000) and Stewart (2000). Throughout the book, we have used various comments and stories from bereaved family members who participated in the research. These are included with their consent and encouragement since all are keen to support health professionals care for bereaved families. Such comments and stories in subsequent chapters are from Dent (2000) and Stewart (2000) unless an alternative source is given. Within such quotes, bold indicates our emphasis of particular words.

Constructions of grandparent bereavement

Stewart (2000) concentrated on the relatively unresearched area of grandparent bereavement. She explored the ways in which grandparents whose infant grandchild had died suddenly constructed their bereavement both as individuals and as family members. In addition, she looked at the ways in which bereaved parents and health professionals perceived grandparent bereavement within the context of the family. The research used a constructivist methodology (Guba & Lincoln 1989) to enable participants to explore their experiences and thoughts in a series of conversations using either unstructured interviews or letters. There were 16 grandparents, aged 54–76 years, of whom 13 were grandmothers; seven parents were from a total of 11 families who had had a grandchild/child die less than 1 year of age. All the parents lived in New Zealand as did 13 of the grandparents, while three grandmothers lived in the UK. The participants were approached via letters sent to three self-help groups in the south of the South Island of New Zealand, and an advert was published in the UK Stillbirth and Neonatal Death Society (SANDS) newsletter. At the time of joining the research, it was between 5 months and 16 years after the death of the grandchild/child. The reasons for the deaths varied from stillbirth, SIDS to illness. Given the chosen methodology and participant group, no claims to generalise the findings are made. However, the findings assist in developing awareness of different aspects of bereavement.

Grandparents viewed the sudden death of a grandchild as an unexpected challenge that needed to be managed both for themselves and their family. The death caused them considerable pain and sadness. Despite extensive life experience, many felt unprepared for the challenge. The focus of their bereavement was as 'parents of the adult parents'. This meant that many placed their own pain second to their desire to help and support the parents of their dead grandchild. Bereaved parents valued this support and the opportunities to share memories of the grandchild with the grandparents. This group of grandparents valued acknowledgement of their bereavement but did not desire ongoing support from health/bereavement professionals. Some grandparents felt that friends, neighbours and society overlooked their bereavement. All the parents and grandparents found different ways to maintain a connection with the dead child, both privately and within the family setting.

A number of grandparents and parents found that telling their stories during the research enabled them to remember and revisit events and ideas about their experience. Several people commented that they had never had the opportunity to talk at length about their experiences. The stories gathered during the research illustrated that each individual constructed a different experience from the same event of having a grandchild/child die suddenly. The research highlighted the value of listening to bereaved people. Nurses and midwives have the opportunity to listen to stories as part of their practice. Instead of minimising this activity as 'I've **just** listened to him/her talking', it is important to acknowledge that this is a vital part of the journey for many bereaved people.

Research into support for families after sudden child death

Dent focused on the support of families whose child (from 1 week to 12 years) died suddenly and unexpectedly from accident or illness. The first retrospective quantitative study (Dent et al 1996) was conducted in seven of the former 14 regions of England and Wales. Postal questionnaires were used to ascertain bereaved fathers' and mothers' perceptions of support, both in hospital at the time of death and in the community during the following months. Although 226 families were identified, only 72 families were eventually contacted. The main reason for exclusion was that all ethics committees insisted that families' general practitioners (GPs) gave permission before contacting the parents. Of the GPs, nearly a fifth did not reply to the letter, 7% could not be traced, almost a fifth of families' addresses were not made available and 15% of GPs refused access to the parents. The reasons given were that the parents were still grieving, had divorced or separated since the death, that some mothers were pregnant or that there were social problems. Under one-third of GPs gave permission, and 14% of families were untraceable. While ethics committees may have been 'protecting' parents, the process potentially took choice away from parents, some of whom may have wanted to be involved in the study.

Of the 72 families contacted, 67 parents from 42 families completed the questionnaires (58%). Therefore, the sample size was not necessarily representative of all families. Replies from these families showed clearly that most parents, while perceiving hospital care as generally 'good', felt isolated and unsupported in the community in the months after the death. Community health professionals in the same study were asked how confident they felt about supporting bereaved families. Replies from 186 health visitors (78%) and 166 GPs (69%) demonstrated that lack of training and confidence prevented them from following up bereaved families.

As a result of these findings, it seemed appropriate to consider ways in which bereaved families could feel better supported and less isolated in the months after the death. From the first study, it was clear that health visitors, GPs and parents perceived health visitors as appropriate health professionals to take on a supportive role. However, lack of confidence and training prevented them from offering follow-up care. Extensive training programmes were not realistic. Therefore, a bereavement assessment tool was designed for health visitors to give a framework for identifying stresses (personal, familial and extrafamilial) as perceived by the parent(s) (Dent 2000). The aim was to assist health visitors to plan follow-up care for the whole family. The tool was developed using a range of literature and research from stress, family systems and bereavement theories.

To test the efficacy of the assessment tool, a randomised controlled trial was conducted in one region of England. Prior to the start of this study, the 23 health authorities in the South and West Region were randomly allocated into intervention ($n = 12$) or control groups ($n = 11$). All health visitors in the intervention group ($n = 796$) were sent the assessment tool to use when they met a bereaved family. This was accompanied by a resource booklet that provided information about bereavement care and the assessment tool. Over the 2 year study period, 184 sudden child deaths were reported. Of these families, 62 were excluded because of study design ($n = 17$), parents not wishing to be involved ($n = 16$) or GPs and health visitors believing that parents would not cope with the questionnaires ($n = 11$). Of the remaining 122 families, 58 were in the intervention group and 64 in the control group. After inviting parents to take part, questionnaires were sent to each father and mother 6 months after the death. The questions related to the support and care given by their health visitors to the whole family, including partners, siblings and grandparents. Responses came from 34 study families and 38 control families. In contrast to the first study, these responses showed that the majority of parents in both groups felt well supported by their health visitors in the 6 months since the death of their child. This similarity could be attributed to the fact that all health visitors were sent questionnaires 3 months before the parents. The questions may have guided the health visitors in the control group to take a more holistic perspective when offering support to bereaved families in the following 3 months before the parents were sent questionnaires. Alternative explanations include the sample size being insufficient to demonstrate differences or that the publication of findings from the initial study (Dent et al 1996) combined with other bereavement initiatives receiving media exposure, contributed to increasing awareness of bereavement care.

Health visitors in both groups were sent questionnaires 3 months after the death of a child. Responses came from 59 (75%) in the intervention group and 51 (79%) in the control group. The majority of health visitors in the intervention group had used the tool and felt that it had been a useful framework to plan care and identify family stresses. They recommended that all health visitors involved with a bereaved family should have access to the tool. This supported the view that a tool, with accompanying information, can assist health professionals to care confidently for bereaved families. The tool is discussed in Chapter 8 and presented in the appendices.

STRUCTURE AND CONTENT OF THE BOOK

The book has three sections:

1. contexts and perspectives of change and bereavement
2. family members' experiences, perceptions and meanings of bereavement
3. professional practice and care for bereaved families.

The chapters develop sequentially through the text but can be read in isolation if required. We appreciate that many health professionals have an urgent need to know about some aspect of sudden child death and will read the relevant chapter. To assist rapid access of information, there are summary points at the end of each chapter. In addition to the reference sources quoted throughout the chapters, most chapters also carry a short list of further reading resources that are particularly relevant to the topics discussed in the chapter. In some chapters we have included questions for the reader to consider. Their purpose is to assist the exploration of assumptions and beliefs about bereavement and grief that may shape the ways in which care is offered to bereaved families. The appendices include resources for family members and health professionals.

CONTEXTS AND PERSPECTIVES OF BEREAVEMENT

The first chapter considers loss, change and transition in the family setting. Families experience many changes. From early childhood people learn to cope with change and transition; these experiences can influence responses to other losses later in life.

In Chapter 2, we explore different cultural and historical constructions of bereavement and consider how these shape both health professionals' practice and societal views of grief. Perspectives of grieving such as stage and dual process models, continuing bonds with the deceased and meaning reconstruction are reviewed in relation to clinical practice. The chapter concludes with Riches and Dawson's (2000) perspective of the resources used by bereaved individuals. This offers a basis for practice, which is discussed in the third section of the book.

FAMILY MEMBERS' EXPERIENCES, PERCEPTIONS AND MEANINGS OF BEREAVEMENT

The middle section of the book represents the experience of some bereaved parents, siblings and grandparents. Although a chapter is devoted to each, the content is interrelated since bereavement is a family concern affecting adults and children. While we recognise that research and theories are important, so are the stories of family members.

Chapter 3 explores the experience of parents and the difficulties they face after sudden child death. These include dealing with their pain, reorganising their lives and coping with changed relationships within the family. Rose's story, with comments from John, gives an account of having a child die suddenly. We also consider the comments made by some parents about support available from family, friends and health professionals.

It is only relatively recently that the grief of children has been acknowledged, and most research on bereaved children has concentrated on the death of a parent. In Chapter 4, we look at what it means to be a bereaved brother or sister, how children learn about death and include comments from the experiences of some bereaved siblings.

Chapter 5 focuses on grandparents, whose grief is sometimes forgotten or overlooked by friends, health professionals and society. Jenny's story uncovers some of the distress she felt as a grandmother whose first grandchild died. Other grandparents comment on the support offered to bereaved parents and the ways that they found to live with the death of a grandchild.

PROFESSIONAL PRACTICE AND CARE FOR BEREAVED FAMILIES

Chapter 6 identifies some of the limitations of existing research as an evidence base for bereavement care and considerations for professional practice are proposed. These are grouped into three sections: recognising diversity in bereavement and grief, defining professional practice with bereaved families, and working in practice with bereaved families. Nurses and midwives can use these ideas to underpin the considerations for practice proposed in Chapters 7 and 8. In addition, the role of other sources of support for families, such as mutual help groups, is discussed.

Chapters 7 and 8 focus on practical issues when caring for families around the time of death and in the following weeks and months. In Chapter 7, we consider the issues concerned in laying the foundations of support for families. These include telling parents of the death, giving parents choices, explaining postmortems and offering information. Support for families does not end at the time of death; this is the acute stage when parents and others may be in severe shock. It is later that the full extent of the death may be realised, and a family has to adjust to life without the deceased child. In Chapter 8, we have concentrated on strategies that may assist health professionals to provide follow-up care to bereaved families in the months following the death. This includes using an assessment tool to plan care and recognising the complexities of grief. The tool was evaluated during the study by Dent (2000). It offers a resource for health professionals and may be freely adapted and copied.

In Chapter 9 we use the ideas from previous chapters to explore the resources that are available to health professionals to assist them to balance the stress and loss that they personally may experience while working with bereaved families.

CONCLUDING THOUGHTS

In this section we have set the scene for the following chapters in the book, all of which are interwoven. While writing this book, we have used the image of a painting to guide our thoughts: a painting which has people in the foreground, landscapes and sky in the background. Each chapter brings a different part of the painting into focus: the family, the background perspectives to grief, the parents, the siblings, the grandparents and then the health professionals who support bereaved family members. This means that we have chosen to bring the family into the foreground for the first chapter. Sadly, it is a place where children do die suddenly.

REFERENCES

Berger P L, Luckmann T 1966 The social construction of reality. Doubleday, Garden City, NY

Dawes M 1999 Preface. In: Dawes M, Davies P, Gray J et al (eds) Evidence-based practice. Churchill Livingstone, London, p ix–x

Dent A 2000 Support for families whose child dies suddenly from accident or illness. PhD thesis, School of Policy Studies, University of Bristol, UK

Dent A, Condon L, Fleming P et al 1996 A study of bereavement care after sudden and unexpected death. Archives of Disease in Childhood 74: 522–526

Doka K 1989 Disenfranchised grief. Lexington Books, Lexington, MA

Guba E, Lincoln Y 1989 Fourth generation evaluation. Sage, Thousand Oaks, NC

Jordan J, Kraus D, Ware E 1993 Observations on loss and family development. Family Process 32: 425–440

Leibrich J 1999 A gift of stories. University of Otago, Dunedin, NZ

Malacrida C 1998 Mourning the dreams. Qual Institute Press, University of Alberta, Edmonton, Alberta

McCall M 1989 The significance of storytelling. Life Stories 5: 39–48

McDrury J, Alterio M 2002 Learning through storytelling. Dunmore Press, Palmerston North, NZ

Nadeau J 1998 Families making sense of death. Sage, Thousand Oaks, CA

Neimeyer R 2001a The language of loss: grief therapy as a process of meaning reconstruction. In: Neimeyer R (ed) Meaning reconstruction and the experience of loss. American Psychological Association, Washington, DC, p 261–292

Neimeyer R 2001b Meaning reconstruction and loss. In: Neimeyer R (ed) Meaning reconstruction and the experience of loss. American Psychological Association, Washington, DC, p 1–12

Office for National Statistics 2002a Health statistics quarterly (Winter). Office for National Statistics, London. Available online: http://www.ons.gov.uk, accessed 1 Feb 2003

Office for National Statistics 2002b Mortality statistics cause. Review of the Registrar General on deaths by cause, sex and age in England and Wales 2001. Series DH2 No.28. London: Office for National Statistics. Available online: http://www.ons.gov.uk, accessed 1 Feb 2003

Parkes C 1988 Bereavement as a psychosocial transition: processes of adaptation to change. Journal of Social Issues 44: 53–65

Riches G, Dawson P 2000 An intimate loneliness: supporting bereaved parents and siblings. Open University Press, Buckingham, UK

Rosenblatt P 2002 Guest editorial: grief in families. Mortality 7: 125–126

Stewart A 2000 When an infant grandchild dies: family matters. PhD thesis, School of Nursing, University of Wellington, Wellington, NZ

UK Central Council for Nursing, Midwifery and Health Visiting (UKCC) 2000 Requirements for pre-registration midwifery programmes. UKCC, London. Available online: http//www.nmc-org.uk, accessed 1 Feb 2003

UK Central Council for Nursing, Midwifery and Health Visiting (UKCC) 2001 Requirements for pre-registration nursing programmes. UKCC, London. Available online: http//www.nmc-org.uk, accessed 1 Feb 2003

Walter T 1996 A new model of grief: bereavement and biography. Mortality 1: 7–27

Walter T 1999 On bereavement: the culture of grief. Open University Press, Buckingham, UK

White M, Epston D 1990 Narrative means to therapeutic ends. Norton, New York

Contexts and perspectives of bereavement

As we noted in 'Setting the scene', grief does not occur in isolation. This section explores the contexts within which loss and bereavement occur. As Riches and Dawson (2000) identified, the cultural and social settings that surround an individual offer resources for their grieving.

The family that surrounds most individuals from birth is one of the social arenas in which people experience change, loss and stress. Such experiences provide the basis for responding to the death of a child. Equally, family members may assist or hinder each other's experiences of change and loss through expectations and behaviours.

Individuals also live in a cultural environment where beliefs, values and practices exist that may shape their experiences of grief. In particular, models and theories of grief developed in the 20th century influence both health professionals' practice and the views of wider society about 'how people grieve'.

REFERENCE

Riches G, Dawson P 2000 An intimate loneliness: supporting bereaved parents and siblings. Open University Press, Buckingham, UK

Family life: change and loss

> No man can reveal to you aught but that which already lies half
> asleep in the dawning of your knowledge.
>
> Kahlil Gibran
> *The Prophet*

INTRODUCTION

The interrelated nature of human life where individuals live within social groups within a society, means that there is no clear beginning point for this book about sudden death of a child. Should we start with the individual or the wider cultural or social contexts within which people live? We have chosen to start with the family because we believe that it is central to the death of a child. Children are born, live in and grow up in families. Families are central to the lives, experiences and losses of many individuals. So it is fitting, having set the scene, to focus on families. Consequently, we develop the ideas presented in 'Setting the scene' and refer to some key texts to explore a range of questions related to 'family'. What, or who, is family? What do families do? Why is family important during loss and change? When, and how, do people learn to cope with change and loss?

THE FAMILY AS CONTEXT

The majority of people come from families. It is where most people start and end life, experiencing many losses and changes between birth and death. This applies both to family members who are bereaved by the death of a child and to the health professionals who work with them.

Therefore, this chapter is not primarily about bereavement or death. Instead, we have focused on 'family' as a social context within which individuals experience, learn about and cope with changes (Fig. 1.1). This means that family members who encounter the sudden death of a child have a range of preexisting resources gained from previous experiences of change. Moos (1995, p. 359) described this in her integrative model of grief. '*One characteristic of coping strategies for dealing with death is that they are typically adapted from coping skills previously used in other crises. Families come to a death with an abundance of coping skills that have been developed over time and with experience.*' We believe the importance of family, as a resource and learning environment, requires nurses and midwives to be **family aware** (see p. 119). By this we mean being aware of the ways in which the family

Figure 1.1

Context and resources of bereaved individuals

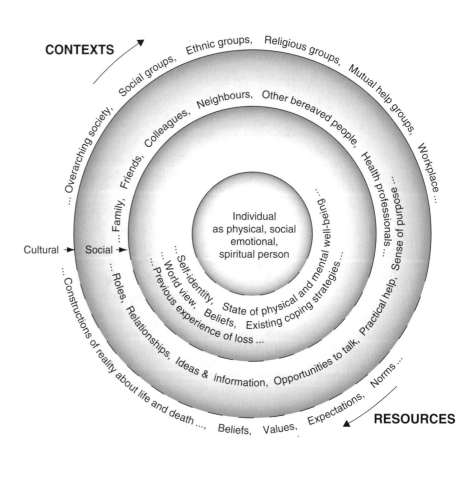

context shapes, supports and constrains the experiences of individual family members. Thus, the individual within the family is the focus of care (Wright & Leahey 1990). This differs from practice which, for some health professionals, is focused on the family as a whole unit (Baggaley 1997). The latter offers a more holistic way to practice. However, in many situations where a child dies suddenly, health professionals may only meet the parents. In addition, health professionals working in a hospital setting may only have a brief time with families around the time of death unless they are subsequently involved in bereavement follow-up. Therefore, in Chapters 7 and 8, we have emphasised the notion of being aware of the ways in which members of a family can influence each other's experience of bereavement.

WHAT, OR WHO, IS FAMILY?

It is said that we are all experts when it comes to understanding the family (Walrond Skinner 1988). Such expertise is generally based on personal experience of family life. This may help us to appreciate the complexity of families; it may also create assumptions about what constitutes a **normal** family by using a reference point of personal experience. Any such assumptions can influence the ways in which nurses and midwives work with families.

Before reading further, take a moment to consider the following questions:

- What does 'family' mean to you?
- Who do you include as members of your family?
- What are the things that are important to you about your family?

CHANGING CONSTRUCTIONS OF 'FAMILY'

In 'Setting the scene', we described our belief that reality is constructed and that knowledge is bound by both time and context. Hence, people may hold different views of what constitutes **family**. In addition, family has the potential to be an ever-changing concept, which is influenced by changes within society. For example, from the perspective of Stone (1977) an historian, 'family' has changed in Western society from the 16th century, when small households were connected to their local community, to the 17th century, when family became an increasingly separate entity. Similarly, Kissane and Bloch (2002) noted that the mortality rates of the 18th and 19th centuries brought changes to family structure and kinship relationships. More recently, Taylor and Field (1993) proposed that the introduction of the National Health Service in the UK changed family structures to become less communal and more fragmented as the state took on responsibility for health care. In addition, economic and technical growth has potentially contributed to distanced family structures, as family members relocate to work in areas away from each other. Changing social attitudes such as the acceptability of divorce, single parenthood and same-sex partnerships have also contributed to a changing view of family in the 21st century.

DEFINING FAMILY

While notions of family may change, how has family been defined, and who makes the definition? A family is conventionally described as a group of persons linked by kinship, which can be established through lines of descent that connect blood relatives or through marriage. Nearly 20 years ago, Walrond Skinner (1988, p. 11) offered a definition that encompassed both the emotional bonds and changing forms of families.

> [A family is] a dynamic, interdependent psychological unit, made up of individuals and the interaction between them, a nucleus of whom form a household over time and may be related by blood or law in addition to their emotional bonds. Whilst a family will evolve and change through the course of its lifecycle, its members will retain crucial emotional significance for one another, of both a positive and negative kind.

Interestingly, this perspective of family makes provision for the inclusion of members who are not physically present in the household. This could be interpreted to include family members who are absent because of distance, separated relationships and even death. The last would mean that family members who have died might still have significance in the lives of surviving family members. In Chapter 2, we explore the idea of such continuing bonds within families.

The perspective of family as a system has become a widely accepted way of considering the family. As Whyte (1997, p. 7) noted, in 1968 Von Bertalanffy emphasised systems theory *as an integrative science of "wholeness"*. As a theory, it has influenced a wide range of disciplines such as social work, family therapy and nursing. Muxen (1991, p. 16) described a family system in terms of connections, where family is *a set of intimately connected people who are mutually influential on each other in some way, and whose relationships evolve over time interactively with each other as well as with the past, present and anticipated future contexts.* From this perspective, family includes people who are important to each other. This is reflected in the commonly used term 'significant others'. Muxen's view, like Walrond Skinner's definition, can also be interpreted to accommodate the evolving nature of family resulting from death, birth and entry of new family members.

So, who decides the people who are 'intimately connected' and thus form 'the family'? Definitions, and judgements, can be made from within and outside the family. From Cheal's (1991) perspective, it is likely that those **outside the family**, such as researchers, practitioners and policy makers, are one step behind the ways in which families exist as part of everyday life. Similarly, Wellard (1997) noted that the nuclear family has been widely promoted in social policy and family nursing models, despite the multiplicity of other family forms that currently exist. As we noted above, a further limitation of using the outsider perspective is that any definition is potentially shaped by the outsider's personal experiences of being a member of a family. The other stance is to consider a definition from an **inside** perspective. In the context of family nursing, Wright and Leahey (1994, p. 40) proposed that *family is who they say they are*. This definition avoids the assumptions of outsiders determining who, and what, is family.

However, it is important to recognise that family is made up of individuals, all of whom may have their own insider view. Therefore, definitions of family may vary according to the perspective of different people. This is apparent in the stories of parents and grandparents who grapple with the implication of relationships with new family members (Stewart 2000). Marie explained her perspective as a mother and grandmother.

> *Family to me is the people that are important to me. That includes my parents and siblings that I grew up with. It also includes their partners and children – that is more of my distanced family. It includes my husband, our children and their partners, children and future great-grandchildren. It doesn't really include the parents and siblings of those partners.*

Rose, who is Marie's daughter, had a different perspective. Her family had extended to include her partner's family members, who did not form part of Marie's view of family. This highlights the overlapping, and differing, notions of family that are constructed from the reference point of different individuals. The other element within Wright and Leahey's (1994) definition is the implicit notion of choice; family says who is family. For adults, it may be possible to make choices, such as re-forming a family by ending a relationship and then choosing a new partner. For children, there are less choices to determine the shape and form of families. The people they live with, and who care for them, may largely determine their family. Hence, being able to choose peers as significant others may become an important part of children's lives.

The changing and diverse nature of families means that nurses and midwives need to be cautious about making any assumptions regarding the nature, or structure, of a person's family. For example, most parents in the study of Dent et al (1996) reported that the health professionals involved in planning bereavement care for the family had never mentioned grandparents. Yet many grandparents offer support to bereaved parents and have an impact on family life. The potential for grandparents to be overlooked is discussed further in Chapter 5.

WHY IS FAMILY IMPORTANT?

Despite varying shapes, forms and definitions of families, the family has been a constant social group across centuries and societies. Most people are closely connected to their immediate biological relatives. Those who are not will associate closely or cohabit in family-like groups (Payne, Horn & Relf 1999). Although there are now many different forms of family, they generally share the common characteristic of committed relationships. Usually, it is within a family that children begin to develop a sense of identity, belonging, expected behaviours and sources of support. During their lifetime, individuals often struggle to balance attachment and intimacy with separation and independence (Walrond Skinner 1988). Human beings need both to belong and to be alone. They have different needs in relation to both, depending on the stage of their lives and experiences in families. So what happens in families? How do they 'work'?

Family system theory can help to uncover the interactions within the family as it adjusts and changes. The theory assumes that the whole is greater than the sum of its parts, which, as Watslavic, Beavin and Jackson (1967) noted, means that a change in one member of the family can bring about change in the whole family. While the application of a mechanical concept to the complexity of human relationships can be criticised, it does offer a framework to consider ways in which families exist and change. Whyte (1997, p. 10) offered the following principles for family nursing based on the work of Will, Wrate and Barker:

1. *parts of the family are related to each other*
2. *one part of the family cannot be understood in isolation from the rest of the system*
3. *family functioning is more than just the sum of the parts*
4. *a family's structure and organisation are important in determining the behaviour of family members*
5. *communication and feedback mechanisms between family members are important in the functioning of the family system.*

We have selected several implications arising from these principles to discuss further. We believe they offer important considerations for health professionals' practice with bereaved family members.

FAMILY AS ENTITY AND AS INDIVIDUALS

The characteristics of family emphasise the interrelated nature of family and family members – the notion that individuals exist within a social context. Each family has the potential to have a separate life of its own. As Robinson (1992, p. 30) described, this is the unique context within which individuals experience, and learn about changes that occur in life.

> *An influencing, organising and creative agent…a living system which is distinct from, yet connected to, the life of its individual members…every family adopts its own unique way for structuring the roles, relationships and responsibilities that direct their family life. They each have their own system for handling life's differing crises, emotional upheavals, conflicts and demands. Families affirm, protect and define standards of acceptable behaviour, values and beliefs.*

Robinson's description emphasised the family both as an entity and as a social group made up of individual family members. The group has shared meanings that create a family reality or 'world' (Hess & Handel 1959). The family world brings a family history that includes expectations of behaviour, beliefs, gendered roles and coping strategies (Moos 1995). These are shared across generations as parents bring up their children. Children, in turn, bring new ideas, beliefs and behaviours, which may challenge existing family rules and expectations and can lead to these being adapted and reconstructed. Hence, as Robinson indicated, the family is both a living and a potentially creative entity that encounters constant change.

Daly (1992, p. 3) described the shared beliefs and values held by families as the '*collective consciousness that is not readily available to non-family members*'. Akin to the idea of a family world, her comment indicates that family meanings, rules, expectations and behaviours may be distinct from, and not accessible to, people outside the family. From the perspective of health professionals, this is a reminder of situations in practice where it may not have been possible to comprehend the ways in which individuals and their families have talked or responded to a situation.

COMMUNICATION WITHIN FAMILIES

One of the central elements to the ways in which families maintain beliefs, values, roles and activities is communication. Communication may exist in varying forms. Nadeau (1998), citing the work of Berger and Luckmann, described conversation with others as a means to maintain, and construct, reality – or a view of the world. Thus communication between family members can sustain shared family beliefs and behaviours. Conversation offers a means to make sense of events and ideas that are part of an individual's experience, by using other family members as resources in this process. While family is an important part of an individual's social context, it is also part of a wider context that surrounds both individuals and families.

FAMILY WITHIN A WIDER CONTEXT

It is useful to consider the surrounding context to the family system. Like individuals, family does not exist in isolation. It has been argued that the family is a sub-system (Treacher & Carpenter 1984). In this sense families are both part of society and part of the local communities within which they live. All of these have particular beliefs, practices and world views, which, in turn, may influence families. This can include expectations about ways in which families **should** behave, bring up children or cope with change. Families experience changes for a variety of reasons. Death, which is the focus of this book, is one particular form of change. However, most bereaved family members will have experienced many changes during their lives prior to a death.

CHANGE AND LOSS WITHIN FAMILIES

Life is inevitably dynamic and changing. Change arises for various reasons that alter an existing situation. 'Change' is a concept, like 'family', that is dynamic and constructed within a particular time period and social context. Change may be viewed as minor or major and range in degree from having a new hairstyle, to going to a new school, to becoming a parent. In addition, change can be viewed as voluntary or involuntary: initiated and chosen by an individual versus imposed on an individual by an outside event or agency. A developmental perspective (e.g. Eriksen 1963) identifies that some changes are expected to occur through the lifespan, such as change from a baby to child to young adult. By comparison, sudden deaths are unexpected, unwanted and create a major change. From the perspective of an individual, and their family, change does not occur in isolation. Developmental changes, such as the birth of a baby, can be viewed both in relation to the life of an individual and the life of a family. This highlights the interrelated experiences of change that individuals encounter as members of families.

THE FAMILY LIFECYCLE

How do families change over time? The family life cycle is one way of addressing this question. It uses a framework of stages that are generally sequential and possibly overlapping, with a starting point of when individual(s) are ready to form a family (Duvall & Miller 1985). A widely used framework, proposed from the context of family therapy, has been that of Carter and McGoldrick (1989, p. 15). They described a six-stage family lifecycle located within the context of middle-class America in the latter part of the 20th century:

- *leaving home: single young adults*
- *the joining of families through marriage: the new couple*
- *families with young children*
- *families with adolescents*
- *launching children and moving on*
- *families in later life.*

Inevitably, reduction of the complexity of family life to six broad stages produces a normative view, located in a particular social context. As Carter and McGoldrick (1989) noted, the lifecycle may vary with events such as divorce and the particular beliefs of cultural groups. Equally, such a framework may not appear to accommodate the spectrum of family groups, which might include cohabitation (not marriage) with children or surrogate parenting. However, the purpose of such a model is to offer a conceptualisation of a complex issue. Carter and McGoldrick's work offers a way to consider concurrent changes within families, which may be valuable for nursing and midwifery practice. For example, ongoing **developmental** changes through the lifecycle can combine with an **unexpected** change such as death. This happens when a developmental change, such as birth of a baby, is combined with the sudden death of an older child in the family.

In addition, at the same moment in the family lifecycle, different family members are at different points in their individual lifecycle. This intergenerational perspective indicates that if different family members are experiencing changes at the same time, then their ability to support each other may be limited. For example, a grandmother who is facing changes resulting from retirement and diminishing energy levels may have a daughter who is raising young children and about to give birth to her third child. The support that the grandmother can offer her daughter may be much less than 6 years earlier when her first grandchild was born. This offers a reminder to nurses and midwives that family members may be dealing with multiple changes within the family at the same time, all of which affect the 'family world'. Concurrent changes, which may be a source of stress, can diminish the resources that individual family members have available to accommodate change. So how do individuals and families respond to change?

RESPONDING TO CHANGE

Change can bring transition, which Golan (1981, p. 12) described as '*a period of moving from one state of certainty to another, with an interval of uncertainty and change in between*'. The notion of certainty could be debated in the context of family life, where frequent changes are occurring. Does certainty ever exist? However, Golan's work does reflect the view that change involves coping and adaptation. The degree of coping may be related to the type of change. Golan used the work of Silverman to identify the diversity of transitions, some of which may be predicted and others may be unanticipated. For example, while pregnancy may be desired and anticipated, sudden death of a child is unanticipated and may require considerable coping and adaptation to move through the transition from life before the death to construct a life after the death. Both the individual and the family as a whole undertake this 'work' of coping. Coping and responses to change are discussed below for the individual, the individual alongside other family members and for the family as a whole. Clearly these are false divisions, since all are interrelated, but it allows several useful issues to be discussed.

The individual

People respond in various ways to change and it may affect any aspect of their well-being including:

- physical, e.g. changes in health
- social, e.g. altered roles, relationships, activities and communication
- emotional, e.g. changing feelings such as fear, joy, sadness
- spiritual/existentialist, e.g. facing questions about life and the world
- cognitive, e.g. finding ways to make sense of the change.

Central to these responses is what the individual is trying to achieve during the transition. This is often described as 'trying to cope with', 'manage', 'get control of' or 'adjust to' the change. Physical changes in well-being may result from the physiological effects of stress, such as raised adrenaline levels. Feelings and thoughts may be centred on how to cope with the change. In cognitive stress theory, Lazarus and Folkman (1984) proposed that change can be viewed as a stressor that exceeds the individual's existing resources. From this perspective, coping can be viewed as '*the changing thoughts and acts that an individual uses to manage the external or internal demands of stressful situations*' (Folkman 2001, p. 565). It involves appraisal of the event and options for coping, which, in turn, affect the emotions experienced and subsequent actions. Coping may use strategies that can be broadly described as problem versus emotion focused and confrontation versus avoidance of aspects of the stressor.

However, the individual does not exist in isolation; their coping responses are shaped by factors such as existing coping style, resources, social support and concurrent stressors. So while it is possible to see how an individual responds to change, the family provides an important social context to this response. Writing about families' grief following death, Moos (1995, pp. 348–349) noted that a '*family history*' of beliefs, values, rules and expectations of the family world can influence individual family members' responses to change. Examples include:

- prior experience, which may have developed rituals and rules to assist the family
- family rules regarding the acceptability of emotional expression
- beliefs, in particular religious views
- gender roles of expected behaviour.

Again, this reaffirms the role of the family as both a learning environment and a potential source of support during change.

So, why do individuals respond to the same change in different ways? For example, two mothers give birth to their first baby. One may predominantly 'see' it as the beginning of a new life, the other may 'see' it as a loss of a previous way of life. One way to explore differing responses is to consider the meaning that it holds for an individual. Adler (1958) suggested that human beings live in the realm of meanings, so reality is experienced through the meaning that each individual gives it. For some individuals, the meaning of change, especially when radical, can encompass the meaning of life itself. The importance of the meaning is highlighted in the work of Parkes (1971). He proposed (p. 103) that individuals have an '*assumptive world*', which is '*everything we know or think we know*'. Change means that in some situations the world needs reviewing and in others it does not. This, in part, will reflect whether the change is desired or expected and the scale of the change. Parkes (1971, p.103) distinguished the different meanings that change may hold in the following description.

> *The life space is constantly changing, novel stimuli, fresh combinations of events, unique communications from others are received and assimilated. Some of these changes fulfil expectations and require little or no change to the assumptive world, others necessitate a major restructuring of that world, the abandonment of one set of assumptions and the development of a fresh set to enable the individual to cope with the new, altered life space.*

As Parkes noted, gradual changes, such as growing older, may enable slow adjustment. In contrast, sudden death of a child can challenge a mother's entire assumptive world. The death brings the primary loss of the presence of the child and secondary losses with changed everyday routines and roles. Many of these losses are located within the mother's experience as a family member. Thus the change creates what

Parkes (1971, p. 101) described as a '*psycho-social transition*'. The death requires the mother to revise her assumptive world, which no longer works. Parents' comments in Chapter 3 indicate the untimely and devastating effects that death had on their worlds. So, how do people revise their assumptive worlds? Parkes (1988, p. 59) identified a need for support and '*assistance in discovering new models of the world appropriate to the emergent situation*'. In this process, family members and the family world may provide support for an individual to find '*new models*' for their assumptive world. This perspective supports the view that family is both the context within which many changes occur and a potential resource to cope with the changes. However, when a major change touches all family members, it means that everyone is trying to cope with change at the same time. As we described in 'Setting the scene', change can create a ripple that extends through the family. Sudden death of a child means parents, siblings and grandparents may all be simultaneously bereaved, trying to cope, needing support and trying to offer support.

Family members responding to change alongside each other

One of the complexities of change in the family is that the same change event may ripple through the family, with each family member having a different interpretation and experience. This may be explained from the perspective that individuals construct reality and make a different meaning from the same situation. For example, the first pregnancy of a woman will bring changes both to her and to other family members. The pregnant mother may no longer be working, which may mean having less money, less contact with work colleagues and being at home more. She will experience bodily changes. She may dream about the future of her child, her role as a mother and the spiritual meaning of giving birth to a new human being. The impending birth also requires changes in roles, identities and activities of other family members. Her parents look forward to being grandparents for the first time and offer to help her during the first weeks after the birth. Her partner looks forward to becoming a father but may worry about being the sole wage earner for the family. Her older sister may not want to be involved in family preparations because she feels angry and confused about this change, having been trying to become pregnant for some years.

The effect of different meanings and responses to change can result in family members feeling alone and even isolated while the family is apparently an entity. Riches and Dawson (2000, p. 3) described the '*intimate loneliness*' of bereaved siblings and parents following the death of a child. While all had been bereaved by the same event, all were '*uniquely alone with their grief even when surrounded by the rest of their family*'. Writing from a family system perspective in relation to death, Wedemeyer (1986, p. 338) commented, '*A death in a family, like any major event, exposes a basic dynamic tension of family systems: it is a **systemwide** event and yet it is also a **personal** event for each individual in the family*'. This tension emphasises that there is the potential for each individual to affect the experiences of other members of the family. As Moos (1995, pp. 354–355) described, interactions between family members may affect each other's experience and response to change.

Family members will naturally interact in a different way with one another. These differences are not necessarily detrimental, but how the members react to the differences may be. An example would be that an emotionally closed-off member of the family may be uncomfortable being around a member who is continually sobbing in reaction to the death. This may disrupt the previous flow of interaction between members, particularly if one person insists that the other's reaction is 'wrong'.

Thus other family members can support, assist and hinder each other in finding ways to cope with change. Consequently, the ways in which families function have been seen as an important context to the ways in which individuals respond to change (e.g. Hogan & DeSantis 1994, Kissane et al 1996). It also indicates that being aware of the surrounding family, which affects the individual, is an important part of nursing and midwifery practice with bereaved people. So, how do families respond to change?

The family responding to change

Writing about loss and death, using information from research and clinical experience, Walsh and McGoldrick (1998, p. 1) proposed that, '*Coming to terms with death and loss is the most difficult challenge a family must confront in life. From a family systems perspective, loss can be viewed as transactional process involving the dying and deceased with the survivors in a shared life cycle that acknowledges both the finality of death and the continuity of life.*' They identified that this requires two family tasks: '*1. shared acknowledgement of the reality of the death and shared experience of the loss*' (p. 7) and '*2. reorganization of the family system and reinvestment in other relationships and life pursuits*' (p. 9).

These tasks enable individual family members to adapt and also strengthen the changed family. This perspective highlights the possibility that members of some families may not be willing to engage in the family tasks and their response may impact on other family members. Similarly, different aspects of the loss situation such as sudden death, ambiguous loss, violent death or suicide may create particular tensions for families to communicate about. So why do some families appear to cope 'better' as individuals and as a family than others? Walsh and McGoldrick (1998, pp. 13–15) identified adaptive variables including:

- '*family cohesion and differentiation of members*'
- flexibility of roles and rules
- '*open communication versus secrecy*'
- availability of resources (family, economic and social) to buffer the loss
- the effect of the loss on the existing functioning of the family, existing conflict or estrangement in relationships at the time of loss.

These variables of family adaptive functioning are identified in other writings and studies (e.g. Johnson 1988, Kissane et al 1996). They offer one way of appreciating the importance of the family as an environment, and as an entity, within which change is experienced and managed.

However, families do not exist in isolation. As we noted above, societal beliefs and expectations may influence how the family copes with change. For example, a perception of societal expectations that 'men are strong and do not cry' may mean that a bereaved father seeks to care for his partner after the sudden death of their child. He may be unwilling to share his feelings and this may mean that his partner cannot find a way to share their experiences and to revise their shared family world.

CONTEXT, RESOURCE AND ENTITY

We have discussed family as an important context surrounding individuals who are experiencing change. Interactions between family members shape each other's experiences. We have chosen to conclude the chapter by focusing briefly on children and change within the family. The role of previous experience in coping and revising an assumptive world means that the legacy of childhood is an important, often hidden, part of nursing and midwifery practice. The childhood experiences of bereaved parents and grandparents can shape their current experience when a child dies. The ways in which parents and grandparents interact with young children in the family at the time a child dies may influence how those children respond to change in the future. Health professionals working with bereaved family members have their own childhood experiences, which shape how they communicate and interact with others. The spiral goes round and round... .

FOCUS ON CHILDREN LEARNING ABOUT CHANGE IN THE FAMILY SETTING

Morgan (1991, p. xv) noted that human beings begin to learn about loss from an early age. '*We tend to assume that the life of a child consists of little more than the gathering of memories that in later years can be recalled fondly. In reality, nothing could be further from the truth. Childhood is, and always has been, a time of trial and loss.*' Examples of trial and loss are apparent throughout life. From the moment of birth babies experience change: leaving the familiar uterus, encountering people and learning to feed. Toddlers also learn to adapt to their changing life: leaving their mother for longer periods, going to nursery school or sharing their life with a new baby. And so changes continue within the family as individuals go from childhood to adolescence to adulthood.

Benoliel (1985, p. 220) emphasised that individuals learn to cope in different ways. '*The template for an individual's pattern of adaptation to loss is laid out during the early years of life. This integrated pattern is made up of coping mechanisms at the biological, psychological, socio-cultural and existential levels that function to support the integrity and continuity of the individual when faced with crisis and change.*' Where do children learn ways to cope with loss and changes? It is parents or carers who have the greatest impact on the way in which children cope with change from an early age. A social environment responsive to a child's needs appears to be important for the development of a sense of capability to cope with adversity and change (Benoliel 1985). Children learn models of behaviour from their parents that may extend into their adult lives. Society, too, plays its part through expectations of what is acceptable or unacceptable behaviour.

Attachment theory, described by Bowlby (1969, 1988), offers one perspective to appreciate the importance of learning about human relationships. Raphael (1984) proposed that the family unit is protected from threats to its well-being where there are secure ties in the family. A child may learn that expressing distress and seeking closeness to a significant other sets off a caring response from that person. Thus attachment and caring can be viewed as mutually reinforcing and the beginning of a lasting relationship. Conversely, in a family where there are insecure patterns, a child is more likely to feel confused and isolated (Raphael 1984). This may be the experience of a child who is constantly changing foster families.

Childhood experiences of loss and the ways in which people cope are clearly remembered during adulthood. Field (2000) undertook a survey of the earliest recollections of deaths held by 54 British people aged 65–80 years. Memories of deaths, which tended to be grandparents and siblings, dated from around the age of 5 years, with many people recalling the effect of the death on their parents' behaviour. Similarly, we have asked health professionals attending bereavement workshops to describe an event in their childhood involving loss (not death) and to concentrate on the feelings they remembered experiencing at that time. Using adult language, all participants were able to recall childhood feelings of loss, which invariably included anger, confusion, isolation, loneliness and frustration. What helped participants most as children was someone who acknowledged their feelings, who listened without judging and who empathised with their pain. What did not help was a dismissive attitude, being left in isolation and having no acknowledgement of their loss and feelings. Such memories indicate the longevity of childhood experiences and their potential to influence future experiences.

If change is an inherent part of life, both within and outside the family, then children cannot be protected from experiences of change. Some of these will constitute loss and bring pain or disruption. Others may be welcomed and perceived as opportunities. Living in a family, with a shared family world, means that beliefs of other family members may influence the ways in which children, teenagers and then adults perceive change. However, children can be helped to feel less overwhelmed by giving them time to talk of their feelings and by acknowledging them so that they feel supported. If children have been taught to deal with minor changes, such as losing a toy, going to school or moving to a new area, then they will have the skills to deal with major changes during childhood and adulthood (Silverman 2000). Health professionals and clinicians have slowly come to realise that the experiences of childhood influence the ways in which individuals feel, act and respond through their lives (Reinhold 1990). Consequently, the events, circumstances and relationships of the early past may have a profound and implacable effect on adult lives. For example, childhood bereavement may, for some people, be associated with adult depression (Raphael 1984). As we noted above, the ways in which family members communicate with each other, and in particular with children, can shape how individuals cope with change.

Family communication and children

Communication in families takes place when adults and children interact. They talk, listen, observe, react to and exchange many sorts of information in many different ways. Talking and being with others can affect how individuals make sense of, and live, their lives. Children take verbal and non-verbal cues from their parents and will act accordingly. Raphael (1984, pp. 114–119), a well-known psychiatrist and researcher, identified the influence that the family may have on children's experience of death. She identified the following types of family response to death:

- *the family in which death is a taboo*
- *the family in which someone must be to blame*
- *the family in which relationships are avoidant*
- *the family in which things must go on as before*
- *the family for whom the loss means chaos*
- *the family that must do the right thing*
- *the family that functions with openness and sharing of real feelings.*

While any such categorisation cannot reflect the spectrum of families, it offers a framework to consider ways in which communication between family members can influence the individual's experience of a change such as death.

Raphael's (1984) ideas relate to death and potentially the concept of 'change' as part of children's life in the family. Some key points can be considered for practice with bereaved families.

Death, and some major changes, may not be discussed in families where such events are taboo.   The family may rationalise such behaviours with beliefs that children need to be 'protected' from such difficulties or that 'life needs to carry on'. The child may be aware of unspoken feelings and secrets, which may increase their fears. There may be expectations that feelings are repressed, which means that the child may learn that their grief is taboo.

Some families focus on finding fault with a family member.   Punishment may occur in various forms of interactions that create a sense of guilt for the child. Such families may be rigid and inflexible, making it hard for roles to alter when change, or death, occurs. Sometimes, there may be a search for someone to blame for the change and children may become the scapegoat, they may learn that guilt is the response to death, or major change, and feel that someone causes these events. The focus of the problem frequently belongs to the family, especially the parents, rather than the child (Reinhold 1990).

In some families, parents may have developed an avoidance of deep feelings.   Parents who have experienced difficult events in their own lives can adopt a somewhat 'cool' attitude. Children may learn from this that they should not get too fond of someone, otherwise there is a risk of being hurt. The family may not seem to be affected by change and members may carry on being busy in everyday activities. This may mean that in a stressful situation a child may cover up their feelings.

Some families deny change or loss and are inflexible about adjusting to different roles and relationships within the family.   In the situation of a death, there may be a need for someone else in the family to take on the role of the deceased. For a sibling, this may mean taking on the role of the 'baby' or the 'eldest'. In such a setting, children may learn that it is wrong to show painful feelings, that grief is not expected and that the family continues as before.

For some families, change means chaos because they are already vulnerable.   Such prior vulnerability can exist for a range of reasons such as illness or previous loss. They may have few personal resources to cope with change and to support each other. There may be existing tensions between family members such as the parents, so a child in such a family is likely to feel even more stressed when a change occurs.

Some families may have difficulty and discomfort managing relationships and change but seek to find the 'right' ways to do so.   Parents learn ways to cope from resources such as books and workshops. They may explain what is happening to children. This may mean that children are supported to adapt to change. However, the discomfort felt by the family may exist at a covert level and may emerge in interactions with children.

Some families have open and honest communication, both positive and negative.   In such families, each member is recognised for his/her own worth and the family has many resources to adapt to change. Children in such families may be able to talk about their feelings and learn that others can offer support to help them to cope with change. When families are successfully able to raise children to independence, the pattern is potentially repeated by the next generation (Silverman 2000).

These ideas offer a reminder of the ways in which personal experience, as a family member, can affect the ways in which adults communicate and cope with change. It must be remembered that such adults are both bereaved family members and health professionals.

SUMMARY: CHANGE AS LOSS AND DEATH

This chapter has identified that 'family' may have different connotations, structures and forms. During its lifecycle, a family may experience many changes. These affect individuals as well as the family system, which may also be affected by outside influences. Children experience and learn about change from an early age both within the family and in the wider social setting. This continues throughout life, as children become parents and join other social and family groups. Therefore, when a family experiences the sudden death of a child, family members already have existing experiences of change and loss. They do not enter the situation as a **tabula rasa**; instead individuals come with resources, as Riches and Dawson (2000) described. These resources include previous personal experiences from within a family and existing resources available from the family. These influence the ways in which an individual copes with and makes sense of loss. After sudden death of a child, family members face living with a change that alters their assumptive world. Similarly, health professionals have personal resources when working with a family whose child has died suddenly.

This includes their own beliefs and personal experiences of loss and families. The challenge they face when working with bereaved families is recognising that their personal experience may be very different to that of other people.

SUMMARY POINTS

- The concept of family is diverse and dynamic.
- Each family is unique; it is a group of people who identify themselves as family, linked by biological and/or emotional bonds.
- Family is one of the contexts within which individuals encounter, learn about and adjust to change.
- A family, in the course of its lifecycle, will experience many changes and these will have different meanings to individual family members and to the family as a whole.
- Nurses and midwives are members of families and need to consider whether their practice may be shaped by personal expectations about the nature and function of families.

REFERENCES

Adler A 1958 What life should mean to you. Capricorn, New York

Baggaley S 1997 The family: images, definitions and development. In: Whyte D (ed) Explorations in family nursing. Routledge, London, p 29–38

Benoliel J 1985 Loss and adaptation: circumstances, contingencies and consequences. Death Studies 9: 217–233

Bowlby J 1969 Attachment and loss, Vol 1. Basic Books, New York

Bowlby J 1980 Attachment and loss, Vol 3. Basic Books, New York

Carter B, McGoldrick M 1989 The changing family life cycle: a framework for family therapy, 2nd edn. Allyn & Bacon, Boston, MA

Cheal D 1991 Family and the state of theory. University of Toronto Press, Toronto

Daly K 1992 The fit between qualitative research and characteristics of families. In: Gilgun J, Daly K, Handel G (eds) Qualitative methods in family research. Sage, Newbury Park, CA, p 3–11

Dent A, Condon L, Fleming P et al 1996 A study of bereavement care after sudden and unexpected death. Archives of Disease in Childhood 74: 522–526

Duvall E, Miller B 1985 Marriage and family development. Harper Row, New York

Eriksen E 1963 Childhood and society. Penguin, Harmondsworth

Folkman S 2001 Revised coping theory and the process of bereavement. In: Stroebe M, Hansson R, Stroebe W et al (eds) Handbook of bereavement research. American Psychological Association, Washington, DC, p 563–584

Gibran K 1980 The prophet. Heineman, London

Golan N 1981 Passing through transitions: a guide for practitioners. Collier Macmillan, London

Hess R, Handel G 1959 Family worlds: a psychological approach to family life. University of Chicago Press, Chicago, IL

Hogan N, DeSantis L 1994 Things that help and hinder adolescent sibling bereavement. Western Journal of Nursing Research 16: 132–153

Johnson J 1988 Cancer: a family disruption. Recent Results in Cancer Research 108: 306–310

Kissane D, Bloch S 2002 Family focussed grief therapy. Open University Press, Buckingham, UK

Kissane D, Bloch S, Dowe D et al 1996 The Melbourne family grief study 1: perceptions of family functioning in bereavement. American Journal of Psychiatry 153: 650–658

Lazarus RS, Folkman S 1984 Stress, appraisal and coping. Springer-Verlag, New York

Moos N 1995 An integrative model of grief. Death Studies 19: 337–364

Morgan J 1991 Young people and death. Charles Press, Philadelphia, PA

Muxen M 1991 Making sense of sibling loss in adulthood: an experimental analysis. PhD thesis, University of Minnesota, Minneapolis, MN

Nadeau J 1998 Families making sense of death. Sage, Thousand Oaks, CA

Parkes C 1971 Psychosocial transitions: a field for study. Social Science and Medicine 5: 101–115

Parkes C 1988 Bereavement as a psychosocial transition: processes of adaptation to change. Journal of Social Issues 44: 53–65

Payne S, Horn S, Relf M 1999 Loss and bereavement. Open University Press, Buckingham, UK

Raphael B 1984 The anatomy of bereavement, 3rd edn. Unwin Hyman, London

Reinhold M 1990 How to survive in spite of your parents: coping with hurtful childhood legacies. Cedar, London

Riches G, Dawson P 2000 An intimate loneliness: supporting bereaved parents and siblings. Open University Press, Buckingham, UK

Robinson S 1992 The family with cancer. European Journal of Cancer Care 1: 29–33

Silverman P 2000 Never too young to know. Oxford University Press, New York

Stewart A 2000 When an infant grandchild dies: family matters. PhD thesis, School of Nursing, University of Wellington, Wellington NZ

Stone L 1977 The family, sex and marriage in England 1500–1800. Weidenfeld and Nicholson, London

Taylor S, Field D 1993 Sociology of health. Blackwell, Oxford

Treacher A, Carpenter J 1984 Using family therapy. Blackwell, Oxford

Walrond Skinner S 1988 Family matters. SPCK, London

Walsh F, McGoldrick M 1998 A family systems perspective on loss, recovery and resilience. In: Sutcliffe P, Tufness G, Cornish U (eds) Working with the dying and bereaved. Routledge, New York p 1–26

Watslavic P, Beavin J, Jackson D 1967 The pragmatics of human communication. Norton, New York

Wedemeyer N 1986 Transformations of family images related to death. Journal of Family Issues 7: 337–351

Wellard S 1997 Constructions of family nursing: a critical exploration. Contemporary Nurse 6: 78–84

Whyte D 1997 Family nursing: a systemic approach to nursing work with families. In: Whyte D (ed) Explorations in family nursing. Routledge, London, p 1–26

Wright L, Leahey M 1990 Trends in nursing of families. Journal of Advanced Nursing 15: 148–154

Wright LM, Leahey M 1994 Nurses and families: a guide to family assessment and
intervention. Davis, Philadelphia, PA

USEFUL SOURCES FOR NURSES AND MIDWIVES

Nadeau J 1998 Families making sense of death. Sage, Thousand Oaks, CA
Payne S, Horn S, Relf M 1999 Loss and bereavement. Open University Press, Buckingham, UK
Whyte D (ed) 1997 Explorations in family nursing. Routledge, London

Perspectives on grieving

> *I learned that when people described their feelings as 'painful' it was not a metaphor. I felt pain beyond anything I could possibly have imagined; pain so searing it raised goose bumps on my arms, made me nauseous, left me panting and wondering how soon I could die so I wouldn't have to feel it anymore. I learned that I could live, work, and love in spite of excruciating pain.*
>
> Mary Semel, after the death of her teenage son Allie in a car accident
> (McCracken & Semel 1998)

INTRODUCTION

Chapter 1 explored loss as part of life. Death is one form of loss that is a certainty of life. Everyone dies and most people live to experience the death of someone with whom they have a relationship. It is, therefore, not surprising that there have been numerous publications grappling with fundamental questions such as 'What is grief?' These have included people such as Mary Semel and C S Lewis writing about personal experiences of bereavement. Such writings offer a different perspective to that of clinicians and researchers who observe and interpret other people's grief. In this chapter, we focus on models, theories and interpretations of grief and mourning. Section 2 includes personal experiences of family members after the sudden death of a child.

The content in the present chapter is based on grieving in various situations of loss including, where possible, material relating to the sudden death of a child. We have included information to assist readers to appraise the context from which the ideas have been derived and to consider the relevance to their practice. This is of importance given that many of the ideas about grief have come from disciplines such as psychiatry, psychology and sociology, which have different philosophies, roles and scopes of practice to those of nurses and midwives. We fully acknowledge that this chapter provides an overview and does not offer the depth or breadth of debate available in some of the resources that we have referenced. Our hope is that the chapter will stimulate nurses and midwives to read extensively, reflect on their practice and advance their work with bereaved families.

CONSIDERATIONS FOR PRACTICE WITH BEREAVED FAMILIES

DEFINITIONS AND VARIATIONS IN LANGUAGE AND MEANING

Some books and people use the terms 'grieving' and 'mourning' synonymously. Others have differing meanings. Therefore, it is important that there is a shared understanding between authors and readers of this book regarding the meaning of particular words. Before reading further, take a moment to consider what the following words mean to you:

- bereavement
- loss
- grief
- mourning.

In this book we have used the following interpretations:

- bereavement is the event or state of having someone die or losing something
- grief/grieving is a person's reaction to the death or loss and includes the process of living with the bereavement.

We have chosen to use 'grief' or 'grieving' as opposed to 'mourning' since many of the families we meet do not talk about mourning. A bereaved mother explained recently that she thought of mourning as '*being the kind of thing that Queen Victoria did after Prince Albert died*'. She did not perceive mourning as part of her own experience in the 21st century. This suggests that nurses and midwives need to consider the words used by others and be prepared to clarify meanings in order to be able to talk **with** rather than talk **past** each other.

CONSIDERATIONS FOR PRACTICE WITH BEREAVED FAMILIES

There are a number of interwoven issues in this chapter. To enable nurses and midwives to consider the points relevant for their practice we have presented a summary of issues at this point in Box 2.1 rather than at the end of the chapter.

PERSPECTIVES OF GRIEF

During the 20th century, a range of writings have emerged from bereaved individuals, clinicians, academics and researchers that offer ways to conceptualise grief. How do such perspectives help to understand why and how people grieve? As in any field of practice, current thinking has been informed by earlier work and writing. In this section, we trace some of the ideas that have developed in the 20th century.

THE RELATIONSHIP WITH THE DECEASED

Silverman and Klass (1996, p. 5) proposed that, 'The modern idea of bereavement began with Freud's (1917/1961a) definition of mourning as the sad process by which "Each single one of the memories and situations of expectancy which demonstrate the libido's attachment to the lost object is met by the verdict of reality that the object no longer exists"'. While Freud's work focused on depression, his ideas have informed other clinicians working with people bereaved by death (e.g. Lindemann 1944, Bowlby 1961, Raphael 1984). There have been various critiques of psychoanalytic theory. Stroebe (1994) proposed that there has been a perceived overemphasis on relationship and attachment with the deceased, without sufficient recognition of secondary stresses such as having to take on new roles and activities as a result of the death. Walter (1999) suggested that interpretations of this theory have encouraged the belief that people need to express (not repress) their feelings in order to grieve in a healthy way.

ATTACHMENT THEORY AND SUBSEQUENT WRITINGS

John Bowlby, a psychoanalyst and psychiatrist in the UK, wrote the *Processes of mourning* (1961) based on observations of mourning behaviour in animals and separation anxiety in children. These were framed in the context of ethology and psychoanalytic theory. He emphasised the importance of childhood events and noted (p. 318) that unsatisfactory responses to loss in childhood, particularly separation from the '*mother-figure*', meant that '*a disposition is established to respond to all subsequent losses in a similar way*' (p. 318). His later work on *Attachment and loss* comprised three volumes with the last published in 1980. This included four phases of grief, with comment about parental bereavement, based on a review of studies where children were terminally ill (Table 2.1).

Box 2.1 Considerations for practice with bereaved families

Perspectives are not absolute truths and cannot be generalised to all *people.* All perspectives offer broad patterns or descriptions of grief without assumptions that everyone will grieve in exactly the same way. For example, models of grief based on the death of a spouse may not reflect the particular challenges faced by parents whose child has died suddenly. Equally, as the comments in Chapter 3 indicate, the grief of parents whose child dies in a vehicle crash may have different meanings to that of parents whose baby was stillborn.

Different theories and models contribute to understanding the complexity of grief. The experience of bereavement can be described and explained from different perspectives such as stress, change, coping strategies, attachment and cognitive processes. Like putting on different pairs of glasses to look at the same object, all perspectives offer ways to appreciate the complexity and diversity of grief. Different ideas do not need to be viewed as contradictory. As Parkes (1998, p. 21) commented '*The important issue is to decide which theory works best for which person and when*'.

Grief is socially constructed. Interpretations and expectations of grief are determined by cultural beliefs and values at a particular point in time. This is illustrated in the differing ways people grieve in different cultures. What is acceptable grief in one culture may be seen as peculiar or abnormal in another. It is also evident in the changing views of grief within a culture: for example, the broken heart style of grieving in 19th century romanticism compared with the broken bonds of 20th century modernism in Western society (Stroebe et al 1992).

Myths, clinical lore and critical appraisal. Wortman and Silver (1989, 2001) proposed that myths have developed in clinical practice. These include assumptions that loss is followed by a period of intense distress and that working through feelings is necessary for healthy adjustment. On the basis of their review, they concluded that a number of widespread beliefs in practice cannot be applied to *all* bereaved people. In addition, unwitting misinterpretations of original sources may become part of practice. For example, Kübler-Ross's (1997) work, first published in 1969, on stages of **dying** has been perceived by some health professionals as stages of **grieving** for another's death. As a colleague said, in an era of fast-food there is an equivalent of fast-information, which uses summaries, factsheets and pamphlets. All assist in gaining information rapidly but generally omit the context of the writing, such as sample characteristics and underlying assumptions about the nature of grief.

Table 2.1
Stages or phases of grieving proposed by various writers

Bowlby (1961) researcher, psychiatrist, UK	Parkes (1972) researcher, psychiatrist, UK	Bowlby (1980) researcher, psychiatrist, UK	Rando (1986) researcher, clinical psychologist, USA
Phases	Stages	Phases	Phases
Protest	Numbness	Numbing	Avoidance
Despair	Pining	Disbelief	Confrontation
Detachment	Depression	Disorganisation	Reestablishment
	Recovery	Reorganisation	

Parkes, a psychiatrist in the UK, extended some of Bowlby's work and published a widely read text *Bereavement: studies of grief in adult life* (Parkes 1972). His observations were based on four studies: the London study (22 widows), the Harvard (US) study (49 widows, 19 widowers), the UK case-note study (94 psychiatric patients) and the UK Bethlem study (21 bereaved psychiatric patients). He described four stages of grieving (Table 2.1). Some of Parkes' work explored determinants of poor grief outcome in terms of physical and mental health. These have been used in texts on grief counselling and nursing practice as a basis for preliminary assessment of the bereaved (e.g. Worden 1991, Wright 1996) and include:

- who the deceased person was
- nature of the attachment
- mode of death
- historical antecedents (previous experiences)
- personality variables
- social variables.

This framework reflects the complexity of factors that are interwoven into an individual's experience of bereavement. Parkes' prolific work over the decades has provided the impetus for clinicians and researchers to explore and consider their practice. This has included various models to describe grief.

DESCRIBING GRIEF

C S Lewis, university academic and author of the Narnia series of children's books, kept a series of notebooks after the death of his wife Joy. They were published as the book *A grief observed* in 1961. This is still widely read as a personal account of living in, and with, grief. Soon after her death, he wrote about his **subjective** experience, *'No one ever told me that grief felt so like fear. I am not afraid, but the sensation is like being afraid. The same fluttering in the stomach, the same restlessness, the yawning. I keep on swallowing'* (p. 5).

Descriptions from individual bereaved people can offer a glimpse into the feelings and ways in which they seek to live with, and make sense of, their grief. Such descriptions and reflections might continue forever, as CS Lewis (1961, p. 50) described, '*I though I could describe a **state**; make a map of sorrow. Sorrow, however, turns out to be not a state but a process. It needs not a map but a history, and if I don't stop writing that history at some quite arbitrary point, there's no reason why I should ever stop. There is something new to be chronicled every day.*'

Another perspective to describe grief has focused on other people's reactions and responses in the weeks and months following bereavement. In contrast to personal accounts of grief, such description takes a more **objective** stance, and is often written by clinicians and researchers based on observations of several, or many, people (e.g. Lindemann 1944, Parkes 1972). Such descriptions indicate the ways in which grief may alter a person's well-being in terms of emotional, physical, behavioural and cognitive changes. Worden (1991, p. 22) provides description and discussion of the '*manifestations of normal grief*', which may provide insights and guidance for practitioners working with bereaved people. Some of the physical changes he describes, familiar to those who experience shock, include tightness of the chest and a dry mouth. He describes a wide range of feelings that bereaved people may experience, including sadness, anxiety, guilt and relief. Worden also indicates that because the normal living pattern is disrupted, there may be behaviour changes altering sleep and appetite patterns. Other behaviours may include dreaming about or seeking for the deceased. Bereavement can also bring altered cognitions with disbelief or a sense that the deceased is still present. For further detail see Worden (1991, pp. 22–30). Many of these changes are illustrated in the stories and quotes presented in the following chapters of family members' experiences of bereavement. Descriptions of grief, whether personal accounts or written by others observing bereaved people, provide insights and frameworks to appreciate:

- the complexity of grief
- the range of changes that a person may experience following loss.

From any such description, the wide-ranging effects of bereavement are apparent. As Stroebe et al (2001) noted, the potentially negative effects of bereavement on physical and mental health have been widely documented in research studies describing different relationships and types of death. The effects have included increased rates of anxiety, depression, physical illness and suicide. However, assumptions cannot be made that all people will experience such responses. For example, Wortman and Silver (1989, 2001) reviewed a range of bereavement literature and concluded that many people experience less distress than expected after a major loss, and some have moments with positive feelings such as happiness.

THE DYNAMIC PROCESS OF GRIEF

Various models of grief have offered ways to envisage grief as a dynamic process of phases or stages where recovery or detachment from the deceased is reached (see Table 2.1). However, both health professionals and bereaved people may use such description as a **prescription**, with expected progress within a particular timeframe (Walter 1999). Such an interpretation does not reflect the flexible intent of the original source material. For example, Parkes (1972, p. 21) wrote *'Grief is not a set of symptoms which start after a loss and then gradually fade away. It involves a succession of clinical pictures which blend into and replace one another ... there are considerable differences from one person to another as regards both the duration and the form of each stage.'* One critique of the stage/phase perspective has been the potential to interpret grief as a passive process through which people pass (Worden 1991). In contrast, Worden (1991, pp. 10–16) proposed four tasks of grieving:

- *to accept the reality of the loss*
- *to work through to the pain of grief*
- *to adjust to an environment in which the deceased is missing*
- *to relocate the deceased emotionally and move on with life.*

The wording of the tasks offers the interpretation that people take an active role managing their own grief. This view has been popular amongst some bereaved people, perhaps, as Walter (1999) suggested, because it suits people who want to **do** something to restore order and control to their lives. Whatever the perspective of grief, there is agreement that it is a demanding and tiring experience. The notion of 'grief work' is implicit in theories such as Lindemann (1944) and Parkes (1972) and in Worden's (1991) tasks of grieving.

GRIEF WORK

The phrase 'he is working through his grief' is relatively familiar in Western society. What does it mean? Stroebe (1992–3, p. 20), defined the *'grief work hypothesis'* as bereaved people undertaking *'work in order to adjust without lasting mental and/or physical health detriments to the loss of a loved one'*. So, is it part of every bereaved person's experience? In a wide-ranging review of correlational and experimental studies, combined with cross-cultural observations of grieving patterns, Stroebe concluded that diverse coping styles challenged the view of grief work as a universal experience. She also commented that it appears to be a concept located in Western society in the 20th century. Of interest is the emphasis that she placed on grief as a cognitive process involving both confrontation and avoidance strategies. She reported (1992–3, p. 37) that *'At some times, for some people, in some situations, working through grief may neither be necessary nor better than non-confrontational or even avoidance strategies'*. This conclusion challenges beliefs that avoidance of the loss is always unhealthy and that expression of grief is a necessary requirement for healthy grieving. So, how do people balance avoidance and confrontation of loss?

In 1999, Stroebe and Schut published the dual process model (DPM), integrating existing ideas of general stress coping theory with premises such as the grief work hypothesis. Coping with bereavement is viewed as having two elements:

- loss-oriented coping, which focuses on the loss
- restoration-oriented coping, which focuses on reorganising life.

The two forms of coping reflect the different forms of stress that can arise from the death of a loved person (Stroebe & Schut 2001):

- the loss of the presence of the person
- the changes that result from the death, such as altered roles, relationships and activities.

Loss-oriented coping includes crying, yearning for and constructing a different relationship with the deceased person. Restoration-oriented coping includes taking on changing routines in everyday life, denying/distracting from the grief and developing new roles and relationships.

Stroebe and Schut (2001, pp. 57–58) proposed that a bereaved person moves (oscillates) between a restoration and loss focus and that whilst the stressors are interrelated, 'Coping at any point in time is either loss or restoration oriented'. For example, when someone is focused on everyday activities such as housework (restoration oriented), there is less opportunity to dwell on the missing person. At other times they will return to loss-oriented coping, such as talking or thinking of the deceased person. The dual process model offers another way to envisage the complexity of grief and proposes that grief is not solely about confrontation of the loss. There remain a number of questions about this model, such as duration of, and triggers for oscillations between the two coping orientations. For example, the manner in which the bereaved move from loss- to restoration-oriented coping may be determined by individual circumstances, personality, gender and cultural background. Further experience in clinical practice and research will offer further understanding of this model.

THE PURPOSE OF GRIEF

Walter (1996, p. 7), commenting on work such as Bowlby (1980) and Raphael (1984), wrote 'This body of work has been widely read to say that the **purpose** of grief is the reconstitution of an autonomous individual who can in large measure leave the deceased behind and form new attachments'. This had been widely interpreted in clinical practice to require ending the relationship with the deceased, often described as 'broken bonds'. However, as Walter noted, many theorists indicated the possibility of an ongoing sense of presence of the deceased whereby a connection or relationship continues. This is apparent in the stories of family members in Chapters 3–5. In 1996, Klass, Silverman and Nickman edited a book entitled *Continuing bonds: new understandings of grief*, which included a variety of research studies describing continuing relationships, rather than disengagement, with the deceased. Silverman and Nickman (1996, p. 349) commented that the bond may continue in various ways;

the central element is '*that survivors hold the deceased in loving memory for long periods, often forever, and that maintaining an inner representation of the deceased is normal rather than abnormal*'; to maintain this bond or connection requires '*the paradox of letting go and remaining involved*' (p. 351). Viewed from this perspective, the purpose of grief is to move on with life, having integrated the death into a sense of self. Edelman (1994, p. 283) illustrated this when she wrote about her dead mother.

> *Her presence influenced who I was, and her absence influences who I am. Our lives are shaped as much by those who leave us as they are by those who stay. Loss is our legacy. Insight is our gift. Memory is our guide.*

In this way, as described in Chapter 1, dead family members may continue to be part of the family through their role in the lives of living family members.

The perspective of continuing bonds does not necessarily compete with earlier theories. For example, Worden has continued to refine and extend his thinking over time. In the first edition (1983) the last task of grieving was '*withdraw emotional energy and reinvest it*'; this was revised in the second edition (1991, p. 18) to '*emotionally relocate the deceased and move on with life*'. His rationale for the change reflects a growing appreciation of the ways in which individuals grapple with bereavement. He wrote (Worden 1991, p. 16), '*It sounded too mechanical, like one could merely pull a plug and reattach it someplace else*'. Similarly, Rando (1993, 1996), a clinical psychologist and therapist, who wrote about the phases described in Table 2.1 has more recently described the six 'R' processes of uncomplicated mourning (Rando 1996, p. 141), which make explicit provision for a relationship with the deceased:

- *Recognise the loss. Acknowledge the death. Understand the death.*
- *React to the separation. Experience the pain. Feel, identify, accept, and give some form of expression to all the psychological reactions to the loss. Identify and mourn secondary losses.*
- *Recollect and re-experience the deceased and the relationship. Review and remember realistically. Revive and re-experience the feelings.*
- *Relinquish the old attachments of the deceased and the old assumptive world.*
- *Readjust to move adaptively into the new world without forgetting the old. Revise the assumptive world. Develop a new relationship with the deceased. Adopt new ways of being in the world. Form a new identity.*
- *Reinvest.*

(From Rando T 1996, p. 141, with permission of Hospice Foundation of America, www.hospicefoundation.org.us, tollfree: 1800 854 3402.)

Is the purpose of healthy grief to achieve a continuing bond? In 1992, Stroebe et al reviewed information on bereavement outcomes of widowers, widows and children whose parent had died. They concluded (p. 1209) that a continuing bond in the form of '*the broken heart orientation to loss seems no more or less conducive to poor adjustment than are dispositions more congenial to breaking bonds*'. Does a continuing bond offer one, or several ways to grieve? A study by nurse researchers (McClowry et al 1987) provides valuable information. During the 2 years of the Home Care for the Child with Cancer project established in 1976 in Minnesota USA, 58 children died. Parents and siblings in 49 families were interviewed 7–9 years after the children's deaths. Three patterns of grieving over time were identified:

- 'getting over it' was characterised by less vivid memories, an acceptance of the death and a belief that it did not affect their current life
- 'filling the emptiness' involved either keeping busy or concentrating on other situations instead of the grief
- 'keeping the connection' occurred when family members had vivid memories and a desire to remember the dead child even while moving on with new activities in their lives.

This supports the view that there are varying ways in which grieving people develop a relationship with their dead child and there are multiple possible outcomes to grief (Corr 1998–9). It also illustrates the increasing emphasis that has been placed on the cognitive aspect of grief, where individuals cope with, and make meaning of, bereavement in different ways. We briefly discussed this in Chapter 1 using Parkes' (1988) theory of bereavement as a psychosocial transition that requires a reconstruction of an individual's assumptive world (see p. 12).

EXPLORING GRIEF AS MEANING RECONSTRUCTION

What does 'meaning' offer to an understanding of grief? It relates to the earlier discussion in 'Setting the scene' and Chapter 1, where we stated our belief that individuals construct a view of the world. The struggles that people face after a significant death include 're-visioning' their changed reality or assumptive world. Neimeyer (2001, p. 4) described this as a new paradigm where '*meaning reconstruction in response to a loss is the central process in grieving*'. Using an analysis of C S Lewis' journey of grief, Attig (2001, p. 38), proposed that grieving has two elements: (a) '*relearning the world*' as an individual and as a member of social groups and (b) a struggle to move from '**being** *our pain*' to '**having** *our pain*'. While meaning reconstruction could be interpreted as solely a cognitive process, Attig emphasised that such grieving threads through all dimensions of a person's life.

- emotionally: feeling and interpreting the pain
- behaviourally: recognising changing routines and activities resulting from the loss
- physically: continuing to live in physical spaces shared with the deceased
- intellectually: questioning why it happened
- spiritually: facing questions about the purpose or uncertainty of life
- psychologically: managing changes to self esteem and identity
- socially: changes in interactions with other people.

In this process, grief is a '*transition from loving in presence to loving in absence. And we reweave that lasting love into the larger, richly complex fabric of our lives*' (Attig 2001, p. 34).

This perspective provides an appreciation of the ways in which individuals construct the same bereavement event in different ways. Braun and Berg's (1994) study of 10 bereaved mothers found that they used existing beliefs and values to try and accommodate their child's death into their view of the world. This is further illustrated in the work of Karen Martin (1998), a former psychiatric nurse. She undertook a grounded theory analysis with 21 American parents of babies who died from sudden infant death syndrome (SIDS), including nine couples and three women whose babies had died 1–25 years previously. She concluded that there are various ways in which parents may accommodate the challenge of the death of their child. One strategy can be to modify the challenge. This means that rather than abandoning an established world view, people change the perspective with which they view the challenge. For example, a belief that 'it was God's will that he died' can be used to place the death within the existing assumptive world. If the challenge cannot be modified, then parents may need to change their assumptive world to accommodate the fact that their child died. This can mean revising beliefs that the world is a fair, safe or ordered place. Jenny described this in her comment at the beginning of 'Setting the scene'. If neither the challenge nor the world can be modified, then people may become 'stuck' between their assumptive world and the actual world where their child died. This can mean being unable to move on by integrating the experience into their view of life.

INTERPERSONAL EXPERIENCES OF BEREAVEMENT

The material we have included so far has tended to present the perspective of the individual in isolation. However, all perspectives of grief have had recognition of the social context surrounding the individual. The notion of the surrounding context and available support is particularly evident in crisis theory. Caplan (1964) proposed crisis theory using public health concepts, such as primary prevention, in relation to psychiatry. The theory is an explanation of situations where people's usual strategies for coping no longer work. Three important features are:

- the outcome to the crisis depends on the interplay between the exogenous (e.g. social resources such as support from others) and endogenous (personal resources such as previous experiences)
- people have a desire to receive help during a crisis
- people are susceptible to others' influence during crisis.

In particular, he identified that families, communities and health professionals can offer exogenous resources to assist people to cope. This has been the premise of many interventions with bereaved people. The idea of endogenous and exogenous factors fits with the notion of resources presented in the work of Riches and Dawson (2000), which we discussed in 'Setting the scene'. Does sudden death create a crisis? For some family members, it would appear to do so. As we noted above, sudden death can bring particular problems. *'Three of the most common include intensified grief, the shattering of a person's normal world and the existence of a series of concurrent crises and secondary losses*' (Doka 1996, p. 11). Wright (1996), a nurse, has written extensively on issues relating to sudden death and evaluated the effects of 100 sudden deaths in an accident and emergency department in terms of the experiences of family members and nursing staff. He has illustrated the way in which crisis theory can be used to appreciate family members' response to sudden death and strategies that health professionals can use to assist them at the time of death.

While health professionals may be of assistance to bereaved people, the importance of family and friends should not be underestimated. They are the people who surround the bereaved. In an historical overview of bereavement research, Parkes (2001) concluded that the failure of many evaluation studies to demonstrate the effectiveness of interventions such as counselling, would indicate that only a minority of bereaved people need them. He offered (p. 42) the view that '... *families exist for the support of their members and, most of the time, they fulfil this function well'*. So, what do family and friends offer?

As we discussed in Chapter 1, the family has a shared world of meaning and members influence each other's experiences. The family environment can provide the opportunity collectively to make meaning after the death of a family member. Nadeau's (1998, 2001) work provided interesting insights about 'family meaning-making'. Positioned as a family therapist who had previously been a nurse, she used individual and group interviews with 48 people in 10 multigenerational families following death of a member. She identified factors that both inhibited and enhanced the process of family meaning-making. Enhancers included frequency of family contact, rituals, willingness to share meanings and the '*in-law effect*' (Nadeau 1998, p. 83) whereby in-laws asked naive questions and touched on subjects perceived as taboo by other family members. Inhibitors included fragile family relationships, secrets and divergent beliefs of members. Strategies that assisted meaning-making included storytelling, comparison with other losses in the family history, characterisation of the deceased by talking about their lives and 'family speak' where conversations '*included agreeing/disagreeing, referencing, interrupting, echoing, finishing sentences, elaborating and questioning*' (Nadeau 1998, p. 157) eventually to weave a family meaning.

Walter (1996, p. 7) noted a similar process to meaning-making in the biographical model of grief. '*Survivors typically want to talk about the deceased and to talk with others who knew him or her. Together they construct a story that places the dead within their lives, a story capable of enduring through time*'. The role of conversations and stories has received increasing attention as a way of making meaning and relearning the world. Frank (1995, p. 53) proposed that stories offer a '*way of redrawing maps and finding new destinations*' for one's own identity. Similarly, Riches and Dawson (1996a, p. 2) proposed that a child's death creates a '*fault-line in reality*' for bereaved parents and that the creation of a mental narrative of events and feelings can help to reconstruct a sense of self. From this perspective, the process of grief involves conversations and stories to recreate self-identity and a new assumptive world without the deceased. Consequently, family, friends and those who knew the deceased are an important part of the process. It also means that nurses and midwives may be particularly important to families whose baby dies around birth; they are amongst the only people who knew the baby.

However, social groups such as family and health professionals do not exist in isolation. As we discussed in Chapter 1, individuals and families are part of other cultural groups, which have beliefs, rituals and practices. These, too, can shape the experience of the bereaved individual.

CULTURE AS A LENS TO EXPLORE GRIEVING

The sociological analyses of Walter (1999) and Riches and Dawson (2000) offer another lens to view grief. Culture provides a context of ideas, values, beliefs, norms, customs and behaviours that surround and influence individuals. Observations that grief varies across cultures (see Shapiro 1996, Parkes, Launganui & Young 1997, Walter 1999) and over time within the same culture (e.g. Aries 1974) support the view that grief is not a stable, universal entity; rather it is a construction of reality that is located within a particular time period or culture. For example, Stroebe et al (1992, p. 1208) wrote of romanticism in the 19th century '*To grieve was to signal the significance of the relationship, and the depth of one's own spirit*'. Such broken hearted grieving involved practices such as wearing mourning brooches and writing popular poetry repining the death. In contrast, 20th century Western society can be viewed as having an '*emphasis on reason and observation and a faith in continuous progress*' (Stroebe et al 1992, p. 1206), that values breaking the bonds of relationship with the deceased and returning to normal functioning as soon as possible.

While it is possible to explore constructions of grief within a society, there is a need for caution since such observations may become definitive statements about the nature of grief in, for example, English or Western society. There may be as much variation **within** a culture as **between** two different cultures. As Riches and Dawson (2000, p. 17) noted, '*Most modern societies are culturally "plural". That is, more and more nations are comprised of [sic] a number of cultures with contrasting conventions, sometimes widely differing beliefs and varying priorities.*'

Cultures within a culture

It can be useful to consider that while each individual belongs to an overarching culture, such as English society, they also belong to multiple social groups that may have gendered, age-related, ethnic and spiritual or other beliefs, values and norms. All of these can shape an individual's experience of bereavement in terms of coping and perceptions of the experience. Therefore, it is possible to describe grief experienced within a range of cultural groupings, such as based on age, gender or ethnicity. It is beyond the scope of this book to undertake a detailed discussion of ethnicity and religion in relation to grief. There is also a danger that such a discussion can identify rituals and practices associated with particular groups that then become expected norms. As Gunaratnam (1997) argued, wholesale adoption of such norms could preclude health professionals from appreciating that rituals and practices associated with a particular ethnic or religious group change over time, and have different meanings for individual members of the group. One group we have included for brief discussion is gender. This choice reflects the widespread statements that 'men and women grieve differently'. What are the possible explanations for such a view?

Gender

Is the nature or extent of grief different between men and women? Focusing on bereaved parents, Lang and Gottlieb (1993) found that mothers appeared to have more intense reactions to the death than fathers. Other studies have reported that maternal grief appears to be of longer duration than paternal grief (e.g. Dyregrov & Matthiesen 1987, Cornwell, Nurcombe & Stevens et al 1997). Mothers might be expected to grieve more because they have had a relationship with the child from the moment of conception onwards. However, does parental grief vary in quantity and quality? Or is it that mothers' grief is more visible to others? Finkbeiner (1996) concluded, after interviewing over 30 bereaved parents, that men grieve as deeply as women. What differs is the ways in which mothers and fathers show their feelings. This perspective is supported by various studies that have highlighted gender differences in coping style. For example, bereaved mothers tend to cry and talk about their experience (e.g. Nikolaisen & Williams 1980) while fathers may be less inclined to talk and are more likely to care for the mother/family and become involved in work commitments (e.g. Mandell, McAnulty & Reece 1980). However, Thompson (1997), with reference to the dual process model, cautioned against the assumption that there are gender-specific ways of grieving, such as loss- and restoration-oriented coping. He argued (p. 82), 'it is a question of degree and emphasis, rather than a simple either/or'. In particular, social expectations of behaviour may create gendered norms (Finkbeiner 1996), which in Western society can mean that men are socialised to control their emotions (Stinson et al 1992).

So do men need and want to express their grief but are constrained by cultural expectations to be strong and supportive? This may be the case for some men. De Montigny, Beaudet and Dumas (1999) found that a number of bereaved fathers desired to have their grief acknowledged by others. It would also appear that other men grieve in ways that are acceptable to them and do not necessarily feel constrained. Cook (1988) undertook a study with 55 American fathers whose child had died of cancer. She named one pattern of grieving 'solitary expressivism' where fathers would deal with their feelings only when they were alone. One father described this as 'my inclination would be to maybe walk out in the garage and sob quietly for a few minutes' (p. 299). However, is a father's inclination from personal choice or shaped by early experiences of expected behaviour? For health professionals' practice, it would seem that universal gendered grieving patterns cannot be assumed to exist. However, as the examples in Chapter 3 illustrate, differences between the grief of individual mothers and fathers can lead to tensions within their relationship.

One final point to consider in the context of gendered grief is the role of women in current constructions of grief. Walter (1999) has argued that in English society, women's experiences of grief have shaped the cultural expectation that grief involves expression of feelings and thoughts. For example, research often includes women participants (e.g. Parkes 1972). The voices heard at mutual help groups, in self-help and published books are predominantly those of women (e.g. Gatenby 1998, Tonkin

1998). In addition, most nurses and midwives providing bereavement care are women. This has the potential to emphasise women's experiences as the basis of 'normal' grief.

Varying popular guidelines within a culture

As Riches and Dawson identified (see p. 34), differing and even contradictory beliefs about grief may coexist within a large, culturally plural society. Walter (1999) identified seven social norms of grieving, which he called '*popular guidelines*'. Walter's analysis is based on white mainstream English culture, which he proposed is also of relevance to countries where people are of English descent, such as in Australia and in New Zealand. The norms do not offer a prescription of grieving patterns, rather a way to consider how people may grieve in different ways. Some keypoints are presented below; for further details see Walter (1999, pp. 138–152):

- *personal grief* represents the belief that people can grieve in their own way, although societal expectations may be imposed
- *anomic grief* describes situations where the lack of culturally determined practices can mean that some people are at a loss as to how to grieve
- *private grief* reflects the belief that grief should be private and not disturb others
- *forbidden grief* describes situations where the loss is denied by others
- *time-limited grief* represents the view that healthy grieving brings a return to normal as soon as possible, with debates about the length of time expected to achieve this
- *distracted grief* reflects the advice often given to bereaved people to take up activities to avoid feeling their loss all the time
- *expressive grief* represents the belief that the grief process requires expressing and/or working through feelings.

It is apparent that tensions can exist when individuals have differing beliefs about the way to grieve. For example, friends ask a bereaved mother 9 months after the death 'Are you still crying?' thus indicating a view of time-limited grief. Similarly, the quote from Moos (1995) on page 14 indicated that family members who believe that grief should be private may have difficulty with another family member who cries and wants to express their grief through talking with family and friends. This can lead people to attend a mutual help group that is, in effect, a subculture '*set up in order to provide an alternative to a mainline culture and/or to individual families in which emotion is forbidden and in which the dead may not be mentioned*' (Walter 1999, pp. 191–192).

If a bereaved individual wants to have their grief acknowledged by others and is offered no such recognition, then grief may be disenfranchised. Doka (1989, p. 4) described this as '*a loss that is not or cannot be openly acknowledged, publicly mourned or socially supported*'. An oft-cited example is miscarriage, where parents may grieve for the loss of their child while friends, family and even health professionals may perceive the loss as an early pregnancy or 'the products of conception'. Comments such as, 'You can have another one' can dismiss the meaning of the loss for the bereaved parent(s). Similarly, fathers' grief may be disenfranchised when people ask after the mother's well-being and offer no acknowledgement of his loss (de Montigny et al 1999). In addition, bereaved family members may lack social support following violent death or suicide because cultural values stigmatise such deaths (Redmond 1996). Therefore, cultural beliefs about the social value of the deceased or the nature of the death are linked to expectations of grieving and the subsequent availability of social support.

THE CULTURE OF PROFESSIONALS

Nurses and midwives belong to a culture shaped by various beliefs, values and structures. These include professional standards, research and social expectations of health care. The culture of the 1990s has adopted beliefs about the need for practice to be based on 'evidence' as opposed to ritual or habit. However, as we discuss in Chapter 6, research can inform decisions about bereavement care but cannot necessarily be applied to all families. Most importantly, there is a need for further research to identify what forms of care suit which people and when. We make no generalisations but would note that some health professionals who attend our workshops do not use research or theoretical writings to inform bereavement care. Instead they search for 'evidence' on technical aspects of care, such as a type of wound dressing, while using clinical lore to inform practice with bereaved people. Walter (1999, pp. 154–155), using the work of Wortman and Silver (1989), defined clinical lore as *'the received wisdom that informs the work of more or less trained practitioners who work in either a paid or a voluntary capacity with bereaved people'*. He proposed that clinical lore in the early 1990s had *'the notion of normal grief (i.e. expressing your feelings, letting go and returning to emotional normality after a year or two) and abnormal grief (not expressing your feelings, not letting go, still in a mess years later)'* (Walter 1999, p. 156). Interpretations of such beliefs in practice may not support family members to maintain a continuing bond nor to grieve in different ways. Clinical practice may even extend to the prescriptive, not descriptive, use of phase/stage models mentioned on page 26.

A process of misinterpretation in practice can also occur when the work of Kübler-Ross (1997) is generalised to describe grief in general. Further reading of her work would reveal that her ideas were based on interviews with over 200 terminally ill patients in the USA. Hence the five stages she proposed described the grief of facing one's own death **not** the grief of surviving family members. The latter receives just three pages of comment in her book. Yet, it is a text that is commonly referred to in undergraduate courses for health professionals. In common with Walter (1999), we find that the most frequent reply from health professionals commenting on what they 'know' about grief and bereavement is 'Kübler-Ross's stages'. It is a reminder that even when research is used to inform practice, health professionals need to be mindful of sample characteristics, bereavement event and underlying assumptions about grief. These all shape the findings and the potential applicability to specific situations in clinical practice. Hence critical appraisal of information is a key component of professional practice.

Clinical lore that constructs a view of 'how grief should be' has enormous potential to influence people's grief through the practice of health professionals. This is central to the debates about normal and abnormal grief. Other descriptors for abnormal grief include '*unhealthy, unresolved, complicated, dysfunctional, pathological, chronic, morbid, anticipatory, traumatic, delayed, chronic, prolonged, exaggerated, abbreviated, inhibited*' (Jacob 1993, p. 1788). So what are the criteria to assign a descriptor such as pathological to someone's grief? Middleton et al (1993) concluded that across a range of theoretical perspectives of grieving, the indicators predominantly used are:

- scores on a particular bereavement inventory tool that fall outside the range of normal
- assessment that intensity or duration of responses are outside the parameters of normal
- failure to reach a designated goal of normal grieving, e.g. acceptance.

As the authors identified, the use of such indicators is questionable since they are dependent on the reference point of 'normal'. This can be constructed by clinicians, researchers and society in different ways and may vary according to different situations. For example, Rando (1986, p. 56) identified that the intensity of parental grief means that '*the normal experience of parental grief so closely resembles that commonly accepted as unresolved, pathological or abnormal*'. Such a view challenges the notion of normal as a universal concept and recognises that it varies according to bereaved groups. Similarly, the earlier discussion of broken hearts and broken bonds indicates that expectations of normal grief can change within society over time. Issues of working with people who may have difficulty grieving are discussed further in Chapter 8.

SO WHAT DOES CULTURE OFFER TO THE UNDERSTANDING OF GRIEF?

The perspective that there are cultural constructions of grief emphasises that the values and norms of a culture can support, shape, marginalise or disenfranchise the experience of bereaved people. Consequently, clinical practice with bereaved people requires recognition that an individual's grief will differ from that of others and from the experiences of health professionals. Nurses and midwives might consider:

- reviewing their own beliefs and assumptions about grief
- appreciating the range of resources which can shape people's grief.

RESOURCES FOR GRIEVING

Grieving is individual. No one else can do it for a bereaved person. So, what helps or hinders people to grieve? Within all the differing perspectives of grief, there is recognition of the resources that assist people to grieve. As we noted in 'Setting the scene' and Chapter 1, Riches and Dawson (2000, p. 16) proposed *'the term "resources" because we want to stress that bereaved people are active individuals, making choices as they deal with their experience of loss. Parents and siblings are not simply victims of circumstances'*. We would agree. Individuals are not passive; they have to do their own grieving. The resources available to them influence the ways in which they cope and respond to bereavement. Riches and Dawson (2000) identified cultural, social and personal resources for grieving. This was illustrated in Figure 1.1 (p. 4) with regard to the contexts within which people live. These contexts shape individuals' grief by offering resources and also constraints to their experience. We have used Riches and Dawson's work to draw together the ideas from this chapter and offer a means to inform the practice of nurses and midwives. We discuss this further in Chapters 6–8.

CULTURAL RESOURCES

These encompass *'systems of familiar ideas'* (Riches & Dawson 2000, pp. 16–17) and include:

- *distinctive, shared beliefs about death, mortality and the 'natural' order of things*
- *general assumptions about the role of parents, the nature of families*
- *descriptions of important social differences, such as between mothers and fathers, adults and children, men and women, experts and lay people*
- *shared attitudes about what is 'normal' and of social value*
- *conventions relating to bereavement, grief and appropriate ways of behaving following a death in the family*
- *assumptions underlying professional, religious or community-based support networks.*

These points identify that beliefs and expectations in the cultural milieu can shape people's grief. The generally accepted practice of having a public funeral offers the chance for friends and colleagues to acknowledge the death and demonstrate their support for the family. Formalised rituals exist within many religious faiths to assist in the transition from the time of death to a changed world after the death. Rituals vary between cultural groups and change over time (Hockey 2001). Lack of conventions or rituals within mainstream society may mean that mutual help groups provide a culture as 'communities of feeling' (Riches & Dawson 1996b), which offer rituals such as the Compassionate Friends' Candlelight Service to remember children who have died. In contrast to cultural practices that may assist the bereaved, the legislative requirements for many sudden deaths to be investigated by the police can cause families further distress. Parents offer some comments about this in Chapter 3. Cultural beliefs can influence whether social resources are available. If an individual has adopted a cultural belief that grief is time limited, will they be willing to listen to a bereaved mother for months or years? If a person believes in gendered behaviours and that 'men don't cry' will they ask a bereaved father how he is feeling? Thus the cultural context influences the activities in the social context of family, friends and others.

SOCIAL RESOURCES

Social resources include roles and relationships that sustain and develop a sense of self-identity (Riches & Dawson 2000, p. 18) and include:

- *a marital or couple relationship in which grief can be shared and the meaning of bereavement discussed*
- *open channels of communication and stable relationships between surviving family members*
- *available groups and social networks outside the immediate family – friends, neighbours, work colleagues, for example*
- *purposeful and fulfilling roles in addition to those within the family*
- *opportunities to become involved in new relationships with other bereaved people or with experienced support 'professionals' familiar with grief.*

In particular, relationships and interactions with other people can provide social support. Aspects of such support include:

- emotional (e.g. caring, being with, listening)
- informational (e.g. advice, information to assist coping)
- practical (e.g. financial or physical activities), and structured activities in the form of counselling.

As we discussed in Chapter 1, individuals generally live within a family. When a family member dies, other bereaved family members may offer support. Support may also be available from people such as friends, work colleagues, mutual help groups and health professionals. Family and friends are often cited as the main source of support for parents (Hazzard, Weston & Gutteres 1992), for mothers (Forrest, Standish & Baum 1982, Riches & Dawson 1996b) and for grandparents (DeFrain, Jakub & Mendoza 1991–2). What does support offer to grieving individuals? Talbot (1996–7) found that perceived helpfulness of friends influenced mothers' attitudes to life after the death of an only child. In contrast, Thuen (1997), in a study of 251 parents from the Norwegian SIDS Society, found that the long-term effects of social support from any source were ambiguous. One of the complexities of any such study is clarification of the nature and extent of support.

Many bereaved family members want support. Even if support is available from family and friends, the bereaved person may feel that their experience is not 'understood'. This may reflect differing cultural beliefs about grief and personal experiences of would-be supporters. For example, Schwab (1995–6) concluded that bereaved parents were more likely to join a mutual help group if other family and friends had not experienced a similar traumatic loss. Such groups offer an opportunity to acknowledge the dead child and share experiential knowledge to help others (Klass 1988, Riches & Dawson 1996b). However, mutual help groups can have their own cultural norms about expressing grief, which means the 'style' of the group will suit some individuals and not others (Walter 1999). Cultural and social resources are interwoven and can assist or constrain individuals' grief. They provide the context within which people use their personal resources to cope with life after sudden child death.

PERSONAL RESOURCES

Personal resources *'help to determine the individual's resilience or vulnerability in the face of bereavement'*. They include (Riches & Dawson 2000, p. 19):

- *a personal 'philosophy' that can make some sort of sense of the death*
- *faith in established beliefs that provide frameworks of meaning that 'place death in a recognizable context'*
- *opportunities to learn from previous critical life experiences*
- *an 'inner-directed' autonomous identity that can distinguish personal boundaries*
- *an ability to acknowledge and express personal feelings.*

The comments of family members in the subsequent chapters illustrate the ways that individuals use personal, social and cultural resources to grieve and construct various forms of relationship with the dead child.

SUMMARY

We believe that the three resources identified by Riches and Dawson (2000) illustrate the complexity of grieving. Like a set of Russian dolls, individuals' experiences are located within surrounding contexts. Grief can be viewed in terms of the inner doll – the personal resources of the individual. These are shaped and supported by living inside the next doll, which is the family and extrafamilial settings. This, in turn, is contained within the outer dolls, which are the culture(s) surrounding family and individuals. Whatever perspective is used to view bereavement, all have the potential to illuminate the diversity and enormity of individuals' experiences.

SUMMARY POINTS

- Perspectives offer broad patterns or descriptions of grief but it cannot be assumed that these are absolute truths and can be generalised to all people.
- Different theories and models are available to describe the complexity of grief, such as stress, change, coping strategies, attachment and cognitive processes.
- Cultural factors will affect the interpretations and expectations of grief and these will change with time. What is acceptable grief in one culture may be seen as peculiar or abnormal in another.
- Assumptions can develop in clinical practice, for example that loss is always followed by a series of stages that must be worked through.

REFERENCES

Aries P 1974 Western attitudes toward death: from the Middle Ages to the present. Johns Hopkins University Press, Baltimore, MD

Attig T 2001 Relearning the world: making and finding meanings. In: Neimeyer R (ed) Meaning reconstruction and the experience of loss. American Psychological Association, Washington, DC, p 33–54

Bowlby J 1961 Processes of mourning. International Journal of Psycho-Analysis 42: 317–339

Bowlby J 1980 Attachment and loss, Vol 3. Basic Books, New York

Caplan G 1964 Principles of Preventive Psychiatry. Basic Books, New York

Cook J A 1988 Dad's double binds: rethinking fathers' bereavement from a men's studies perspective. Journal of Contemporary Ethnography 17: 285–308

Cornwell J, Nurcombe B, Stevens L 1977 Family response to loss of a child by sudden infant death syndrome. Medical Journal of Australia 1: 656–658

Corr C 1998–9 Enhancing the concept of disenfranchised grief. OMEGA, Journal of Death and Dying 38: 1–20

de Montigny F, Beaudet L, Dumas L 1999 A baby has died: the impact of perinatal loss on family social networks. Journal of Obstetric, Gynaecology and Neonatal Nursing 28: 151–155

DeFrain J, Jakub D, Mendoza B 1991–2 The psychological effects of sudden infant death on grandmothers and grandfathers. OMEGA, Journal of Death and Dying 24: 165–182

Doka K 1989 Disenfranchised grief. Lexington Books, Lexington, MA

Doka K 1996 Sudden loss: the experiences of bereavement. In: Doka K (ed) Living with grief after sudden loss. Taylor & Francis, Philadelphia, PA, p 11–15

Dyregrov A, Matthiesen SB 1987 Similarities and differences in mothers' and fathers' grief following the death of an infant. Scandinavian Journal of Psychology 28: 1–15

Edelman H 1994 Motherless daughters. Hodder Stoughton, Australia

Finkbeiner A 1996 After the death of a child. Living with loss through the years. Johns Hopkins University Press, Baltimore, MD

Forrest G, Standish E, Baum J 1982 Support after perinatal death: a study of support and counselling after perinatal bereavement. British Medical Journal, 285: 1475–1479

Frank A 1995 The wounded storyteller. University of Chicago Press, Chicago, IL

Gatenby B 1998 For the rest of our lives after the death of a child. Reed Books, Auckland, NZ

Gunaratnam Y 1997 Culture is not enough: a critique of multi-culturalism in palliative care. In: Field D, Hockey J, Small N (eds) Death, gender and ethnicity. Routledge, London, p 166–186

Hazzard A, Weston J, Gutteres C 1992 After a child's death: factors related to parental bereavement. Journal of Development and Behavioural Paediatrics 13: 24–30

Hockey J 2001 Changing death rituals. In Hockey J, Katz J, Small N (eds) Grief mourning and death ritual. Open University Press, Buckingham, UK, p 185–211

Jacob S 1993 An analysis of the concept of grief. Journal of Advanced Nursing 18: 1787–1794

Klass D 1988 Parental grief: Solace and resolution. Springer, New York

Klass D, Silverman S, Nickman S (eds) 1996 Continuing bonds. New understandings of grief. Taylor & Francis, Washington, DC

Kübler-Ross E 1997 On death and dying. Touchstone, New York

Lang A, Gottlieb L 1993 Parental grief reactions and marital intimacy following infant death. Death Studies 17: 233–255

Lewis CS 1961 A grief observed. Harper Collins, New York

Lindemann E 1944 Symptomatology and management of acute grief. American Journal of Psychiatry 101: 141–148

Mandell F, McAnulty EH, Reece RM 1980 Observations of paternal response to sudden unanticipated infant death. Pediatrics 72: 652–657

Martin K 1998 When a baby dies of SIDS: the parents' grief and search for reason. Qual Institute Press, University of Alberta, Edmonton, Alberta

McClowry S, Davies E, May K et al 1987 The empty space phenomenon. Death Studies 11: 361–374

McCraken A, Semel M (eds) 1998 A broken heart still beats: after your child dies. Hazelden, Center City, MN

McGreal D, Evans BJ Burrows GD 1997 Gender differences in coping following loss of a child through miscarriage or stillbirth: a pilot study. Stress Medicine 13: 159–165

Middleton W, Raphael B, Martinek N et al 1993 Pathological grief reactions. In: Stroebe M, Stroebe W, Hansson R (eds) The handbook of bereavement: theory, research and intervention. Cambridge University Press, New York, p 44–61

Moos N 1995 An integrative model of grief. Death Studies 19: 337–364

Nadeau J 1998 Families making sense of death. Sage, Thousand Oaks, CA

Nadeau J 2001 Family construction of meaning. In: Neimeyer R (ed) Meaning reconstruction and the experience of loss. American Psychological Association, Washington, DC, p 95–112

Neimeyer R 2001 Meaning reconstruction and loss. In: Neimeyer R (ed) Meaning reconstruction and the experience of loss. American Psychological Association, Washington, DC, p 1–12

Nikolaisen S, Williams R 1980 Parents' views of support following the loss of their infant to SIDS. Western Journal of Nursing Research 2: 593–560

Parkes C 1972 Bereavement: studies in grief in adult life. Tavistock, London

Parkes C 1988 Bereavement as a psychosocial transition: processes of adaptation to change. Journal of Social Issues 44: 53–65

Parkes C 1998 Traditional models and theories of grief. Bereavement Care 17: 21–23

Parkes C 2001 A historical overview of the scientific study of bereavement. In: Stroebe M, Hansson R, Stroebe W et al (eds) Handbook of bereavement research. American Psychological Association, Washington, DC, p 25–45

Parkes C, Launganui P, Young B (eds) 1997 Death and bereavement across cultures. Routledge, London

Rando T 1986 Parental bereavement: an exception to the general conceptualisations of mourning. In: Rando T (ed) Parental loss of a child. Research Press, Champaign IL, p 45–58

Rando T 1993 Treatment of complicated mourning. Research Press, Champaign, IL

Rando T 1996 Complications in mourning traumatic death. In: Doka K (ed) Living with grief after sudden loss. Taylor & Francis, Philadelphia, PA, p 139–159

Raphael B 1984 The anatomy of bereavement, 3rd edn. Unwin Hyman, London

Redmond L 1996 Sudden violent death. In: Doka K (ed) Living with grief after sudden loss. Taylor & Francis, Philadelphia, PA, p 53–73

Riches G, Dawson P 1996a 'An intimate loneliness': evaluating the impact of a child's death on parental self-identity and marital relationships. Journal of Family Therapy 18: 1–22

Riches G, Dawson P 1996b Communities of feeling: the culture of bereaved families. Mortality 1: 143–161

Riches G, Dawson P 2000 An intimate loneliness: supporting bereaved parents and siblings. Open University Press, Buckingham, UK

Schwab R 1995–6 Bereaved parents and support group participation. OMEGA, Journal of Death and Dying 32: 49–61

Shapiro E 1996 Family bereavement and cultural diversity: a social developmental perspective. Family Process 35: 313–332

Silverman P, Klass D 1996 Introduction: what's the problem? In: Klass D, Silverman P, Nickman S (eds) Continuing bonds. New understandings of grief. Taylor & Francis, Philadelphia, PA, p 3–23

Silverman P, Nickman S 1996 Concluding thoughts. In: Klass D, Silverman P, Nickman S (eds) Continuing bonds. New understandings of grief. Taylor & Francis, Philadelphia, PA, p 349–355

Stinson K, Lasker J, Lohmann J et al 1992 Parents' grief following pregnancy loss: a comparison of mothers and fathers. Family Relations 41: 218–23

Stroebe MS 1992–3 Coping with bereavement: a review of the grief work hypothesis. OMEGA, Journal of Death and Dying 26: 19–42

Stroebe M 1994 The broken heart phenomenon: an examination of the mortality of bereavement. Journal of Community and Applied Social Psychology 4: 47–61

Stroebe M, Schut H 1999 The dual process model of coping with bereavement: rationale and description. Death studies 23(3): 197–224

Stroebe M, Schut H 2001 Meaning making in the dual process of coping with bereavement. In: Neimeyer R (ed) Meaning reconstruction and the experience of loss. American Psychological Association, Washington, DC, p 55–75

Stroebe M, Gergen M, Gergen K et al 1992 Broken hearts or broken bonds. Love and death in historical perspective. American Psychologist 47: 1205–1212

Stroebe M, Hansson R, Stroebe W et al 2001 Introduction: concepts and issues in contemporary research on bereavement. In Stroebe M, Hansson R, Stroebe W et al (eds) Handbook of bereavement research. American Psychological Association, Washington, DC, p 3–22

Talbot K 1996–7 Mothers now childless: survival after the death of an only child. OMEGA, Journal of Death and Dying 34: 177–189

Thompson N 1997 Masculinity and loss. In: Field D, Hockey J, Small N (eds) Death, gender and ethnicity. Routledge, London, p 76–88

Thuen F 1997 Social support after the loss of an infant child: a long-term perspective. Scandinavian Journal of Psychology 38: 103–110

Tonkin L 1998 Still life. Hazard Press, Christchurch, NZ

Walter T 1996 A new model of grief: bereavement and biography. Mortality 1: 7–27

Walter T 1999 On bereavement: the culture of grief. Open University Press, Buckingham, UK

Worden JW 1983 Grief counselling and grief therapy. Tavistock, London

Worden JW 1991 Grief counselling and grief therapy, 2nd edn. Routledge, London

Wortman C, Cohen Silver R 1989 The myths of coping with loss. Journal of Consulting and Clinical Psychology 57: 349–357

Wortman C, Silver R 2001 The myths of coping with loss revisited. In Stroebe M, Hansson R, Stroebe W et al (eds) Handbook of bereavement research. American Psychological Association, Washington, DC, p 405–429

Wright B 1996 Sudden death, 2nd edn. Churchill Livingstone, Edinburgh

USEFUL SOURCES FOR NURSES AND MIDWIVES

Field D, Hockey J, Small N (eds) 1997 Death, gender and ethnicity. Routledge, London

Hockey J, Katz J, Small N (eds) 2001 Grief, mourning and death ritual Open University Press, Buckingham UK

Walter T (1999) On bereavement: the culture of grief. Open University Press, Buckingham, UK

Family members' experiences, perceptions and meanings of bereavement

What happens to parents when they can no longer hold a child in their arms or they lose their hopes and dreams for the future? What do siblings feel after the sudden death of a brother or sister? How do grandparents grieve while witnessing the pain and powerlessness of their own sons or daughters? What impact does the death have on relationships within the family and what effect do others outside the family have? These are just a few questions that are illuminated through the stories and comments of family members in the next three chapters. The content does not provide a definitive perspective about 'how parents, siblings or grandparents grieve'. Rather it reflects some of the issues and ways in which individuals experience, perceive and make a meaning from the death. Consequently, the chapters are about diversity.

Family bereavement: learning from parents

> *When a child dies, we lose part of ourselves as parents, part of our past and an enormous part of our future. Dreams are shattered. We miss our children physically and emotionally, minute by minute and in the following years that seem to stretch without end, as time becomes a test of endurance. We may question the spiritual beliefs we have held all our lives. The relationships we took for granted with our family and friends may change. These changes seem to pile up on that one original loss.*
>
> Bev Gatenby
> *1998, whose daughter Rose died*

INTRODUCTION

The comment from Bev Gatenby offers an insight into the meaning that the sudden and unexpected death of a child has for a parent. She describes the life-changing effects such a death meant for her. In addition, such grief is not solely individual; the bereavement brings changes to existing relationships with the surrounding social context of family and friends. This section on family bereavement begins by considering the experience of bereaved parents. All parents have a story to tell of their child's death, one they know and remember well even when the event occurred many years before (Peppers & Knapp 1980). This chapter considers the grief of parents, differences between the grief of mothers and fathers, parents' experience of helping surviving children, and the social resources that are available to them in the months following the death. The experiences of siblings and grandparents are explored in subsequent chapters.

THE CONTEXT OF THIS CHAPTER

This chapter begins with the story of Rose whose daughter Ruby died unexpectedly, 9 days after birth, because of a rare congenital condition (Box 3.1). Rose included her perspective of the impact that Ruby's death had on her partner, John. Like several other fathers we approached, John decided that he could not write about his experience. However, he did read, comment and share some of his thoughts with Rose as she wrote this story. To expand the discussion in this chapter we have used quotations from Stewart (2000) and Dent (2000). Quotations from parents derived from other sources are acknowledged; these have been cited particularly in the sensitive work of Sarnoff Schiff (1977), Riches and Dawson (2000), Rosenblatt (2000) and Silverman (2000). Throughout, we have emphasised that grief is diverse and that there are differences within, as well as between, gendered groups. We have indicated, where possible, whether fathers or mothers made the comments. As we discussed in earlier chapters, people find different ways of grieving. Therefore, this chapter does not claim that all bereaved parents will grieve in the same way; it offers insights into some parents' experiences.

Box 3.1 Rose's story, with comments from John, about Ruby's death

At the time of Ruby's death, John and I seemed quite similar in the way we dealt with things – in the way we talked with our other two daughters and what we wanted at Ruby's funeral. However, I did notice that when friends came around to offer sympathy John would go and sit in the bedroom. After this had happened a few times I asked him why. He said he felt left out of the grief – like people seemed to focus only on me as the mother. When I thought about it I realised that it was true – maybe this only happens when it is the death of a baby. One of the things that really helped me come to terms with Ruby's death was writing poems. This was not something I had done since leaving high school but it just seemed to come out. John loved to read them and he said that they were just how he felt too. I guess they helped him a little too, just by reading them. It was a great relief for me to be able to join the Baby Bereavement Group soon after Ruby's death – having a place when it was okay to cry or get angry – no-one looked at me funny or told me it was time to get back to normal. I believe that is one of the major differences in our coping styles.

Box 3.1
Continued

I like to talk about how I am feeling. John keeps it very much to himself. Even now, nearly 8 years later, I am happy to talk about any aspects surrounding Ruby's birth, short life and death, whereas John prefers not to talk about it at all.

When I look back at what happened during those 9 days, I can now say that I no longer feel any guilt – I know that I did everything that I possibly could to help her. I also believe that the care she received was the best that could be given. There are one or two issues centred on the time of her death, and immediately after that, which I was not happy about but I have come to terms with them now. I no longer feel angry and, because I know there is nothing I can do to change them, I can let them go. Although it seems a strange thing to say, I have had so many good things come out of the tragedy of Ruby's death. My life took a new direction and I have found great pleasure in the way my life has developed.

The decision on whether or not to attempt another pregnancy was too hard so we left it in God's hands. Being 40 years old at the time of Ruby's death meant that I needed to become pregnant fairly quickly. Four months after Ruby died, I became pregnant. Right from the start we decided not to have an amniocentesis test. We had had one with Ruby and it had not been a pleasant experience. The test couldn't diagnose the condition that Ruby died from. So we could see no point. We had the routine scans and found out that I was carrying a boy. This caused mixed feelings. I knew that John was happy – we had always wanted a son and had been slightly disappointed when we found out that Ruby wasn't a boy. Other people's reactions were interesting as well. So many people thought, and said, that it was great that we were having a boy and felt that it would somehow be a real compensation for Ruby dying. I had an uncomplicated (physically) pregnancy, but emotionally I was torn. I really longed to have this baby but I was scared of another 'failure'. I often ignored the fact that I was pregnant and I often think that I short changed Nathan by not being as involved in the pregnancy. We had lots of discussions with our doctor about precautions we could take to try and ensure an uncomplicated delivery with a baby who would live. In the end we knew that if Nathan was born with the same problem as Ruby, then no medical cure was available. We were told that genetically we had a 1 in 4 chance of the same thing recurring. I settled on some very illogical statistics of my own. As Nathan was our fourth child and we had already had two without any problems and one with, he would be fine. Ruby was our 1 in 4. I was, of course, right. Nathan is now a perfectly healthy, noisy and very active 6 year old. He, along with my ability to write poetry and my new direction in life, is a gift from Ruby.

Box 3.1
Continued

As the years have passed, the pain has diminished. However we have had one major setback. When the scandal of organ retention hit the news it was like a blow to the chest. It seemed to fire us straight back into the past with all its associated pain, disbelief and anger. At the time of Ruby's death we were rung by someone from the coroner's office and asked if a sample could be taken of her heart and lungs in order to reach a proper diagnosis of cause of death. Because we were waiting to take her body home and we were booked on a flight it meant that there was only about 24 hours to perform the autopsy and release her body. We agreed and duly went home to do what we had to do. It was a couple of weeks later that we received a letter from the School of Medicine thanking us for the donation of Ruby's heart and lungs. We were shocked. That was not what we had agreed to, and I did attempt to follow it up. Unfortunately, I was also caught up in another dispute about why I had been sent a questionnaire from a research study that asked about the sleeping and eating patterns of my baby – who was dead. So I didn't have the energy to sort both things. I didn't get round to chasing up the School of Medicine after they didn't answer my letter and the matter just dropped out of my mind. I had not realised that believing that Ruby had not been buried intact had been a big issue for John. It took a long time and several phone calls, some from our doctor and one from John's psychiatrist, before we finally heard from the School of Medicine that the original letter had been a mistake and that they had only taken small biopsies of Ruby's heart and lungs. The good thing that came out of this for us was John finally being able to put some of his anger to rest.

PARENTS' GRIEF

Rose's story uncovers some of the ways in which Ruby's death has changed her life and she reveals the challenge that it presented to herself and her family. As Rando (1986, p. 6) wrote, '*The loss of a child through death is not quite like any other loss known. Ask adults what they dread most and the majority will state that, while they worry about the loss of a parent, spouse, sibling or friend, the loss they fear they could never cope with, is the death of their child.*' When a child dies unexpectedly, the death ends the world in which the parents have lived (Brice 1991a,b) so that they can no longer rely on the major assumptions that they have made about themselves and the world (Gilbert & Smart 1992). They enter a new world in which they may have little understanding of the child's dying and death and how to react to it (Rosenblatt 2000). In particular, the sudden death of a child challenges the order of the expected world where parents predecease their children. As Rando (1986, p. 10) described, death of a child is a threat to the parental role.

Parents take on the roles of protector, provider and problem-solver. They become accustomed to being self-sufficient and in control of what happens to and for the child. Parents become used to being able to 'fix' things so they will work to the child's advantage. The broken bicycle is repaired, the upset feelings after a friend's rejection are soothed. These daily interactions in successfully caring for the child serve to define the parents' senses of self, role, and identity.

The event can precipitate a crisis of emotion and experience that is devastating as well as pervasive for parents (Lehman et al 1989). Parents' reactions to such an event can take many forms. The distress of present-day parents may be heightened because many lack cultural patterns of behaviour and rituals to help them to cope with, and make meaning of, what has happened (Mulkay 1993).

Death may come at a point when parents are engaged in tasks of raising a family, juggling work and family obligations and trying to establish themselves as adults (Gilbert & Smart 1992). The meaning that the death represents will also be shaped by the circumstances of death and the relationship and attachment the parent had with their child. In particular, the circumstances of death may influence the support available to parents. For example, when a woman has a miscarriage, the baby is not visible or known. She may grieve intensely and yet her pain may not be recognised and may be compounded by unhelpful comments denigrating her loss, such as 'It was **only** a miscarriage'. In contrast, the death of a young infant following accident, illness or sudden infant death syndrome (SIDS) is the death of a visible child. Yet it may cause some bystanders to wonder why such a short life should cause prolonged and intense grief for parents. There may be greater recognition by others of the death of an older child, who has developed a personality and whose activities leave many memories behind. However, there is no guarantee that support for such parents is more forthcoming. When a child has died from murder, manslaughter or from suicide, the parents may also face shunning by others because of the stigma associated with such deaths (Redmond 1996, Stillion 1996). Whatever the circumstances, the unexpectedness of being told of the death of their child is a shattering experience.

PARENTS' EXPERIENCE AROUND THE TIME OF DEATH

BEING TOLD OF THE DEATH

One of the life-changing moments that any parent faces is hearing the news of their child's death. Dent et al (1996) found that a doctor spoke to the majority of parents to confirm the death of their child. Most parents were able to recall the words used and only a small proportion (4%) would have preferred to be told in a different way. Over half the parents said how well it had been done and appreciated the difficulty of the task and the sensitive way the doctors dealt with it.

They were very caring. It must have been a hard thing to do. They really did care, which always helps.

We were told very, very sensitively by the doctor in charge, told with some emotion and sadness, which helped us enormously.

At first the doctor was very helpful as he took us into a private room and told us what the illness was, and that our son would die. This was good as he didn't want to build up our hopes too much. All in all, he was a very caring considerate doctor.

These comments are encouraging and are similar to those found in a UK study of parental views about care at the time their child died (Finlay & Dallimore 1991). The authors found that over half of the parents who had been told by doctors or nurses felt that the interview had been handled reasonably or sympathetically. In such a situation, one of the immediate questions that parents have is 'Why, or how, did my child die?'

THE CAUSE AND NATURE OF DEATH

The cause and nature of death may be a major factor in the meaning the loss holds for parents. For most, if not all parents, the cause of death is an important piece of information (Rosenblatt 2000). This is illustrated in the title of Martin's work (1998) with American SIDS parents, *Searching for reason.*

KNOWING A CAUSE OF DEATH

In some situations, such as miscarriage or SIDS, the physical cause of death may not be known. Dent et al (1996) found that parents felt distressed that there was no medical explanation for the cause of death.

There weren't any answers to his death. There wasn't anything wrong with him. He was a happy healthy toddler.

The questions were answered but I could not say that I was satisfied. This is because nobody could answer the question why our baby died.

No physical or medical reason – only SIDS, which only means that my son died. No real satisfaction.

We didn't really have a reason why [name] died. The doctor at the hospital thought it was one thing, our GP thought it was something else.

The lack of specified cause for the death can mean that parents are constantly seeking for a reason over the years. Therefore, when new theories of SIDS are described in the media, parents may go back to reanalyse the death to see if this reason could account for it. In Rosenblatt's study (2000), parents engaged in a great deal of detective work to find a cause. This included consultation with genetics experts or close inspection of the accident scene. If the death was accidental, the parents' story included an account of how or why the accident came to happen. Linked to the cause of death is the nature of death, which also shapes parents' experiences of bereavement. Space constraints preclude comment on the nature of all the various circumstances of death where a child may die suddenly and unexpectedly. We have selected three for brief comment, where the circumstances may mean that parents receive limited support from others: miscarriage, homicide and suicide. Further reading about other situations in which parents are bereaved is listed at the end of the chapter.

Miscarriage

Miscarriage can have varying meanings for parents. The meaning is linked to the parent–child relationship, which develops with varying intensity during pregnancy for most mothers and many fathers. Miscarriage may mean the loss of hopes, dreams and expectations invested in the hoped-for child, with whom an attachment is already developing. The miscarriage may challenge parental self-identity. Are they still 'really' parents if their child was not fully developed or alive? Some mothers may derive consolation from having conceived; others may experience fears about their fertility and have a sense of vulnerability (Mander 1994). As we mentioned above, other people may dismiss such a loss. The parents' grief may be disenfranchised (see p. 36) because to the outsider there was no visible child.

For some parents, the miscarriage may not represent a distressing loss. One mother, who miscarried at 17 weeks after 7 weeks of bleeding, described her experience in the following words (Moulder 2001, pp. 107–108): '*It was relief rather than grief. I don't think I ever grieved for it. I wasn't ever aware that I was carrying a baby. I never got upset about it at all. I shed no tears and I normally cry quite easily.*'

Homicide

Unexpected, violent or difficult deaths, which include homicide, have a number of consequences for bereaved family members. They may give rise to strong emotions, intrusive thoughts and affect future social relationships (Riches & Dawson 2000, p. 105). In addition, grief may become entangled with experiences in the criminal justice system (Redmond 1996). The reality of the situation may be hard to grasp, as a father explained (Silverman 2000, p. 132):

> *When you first hear, your response is to block it out, and to pretend that everyone is wrong, that there is a terrible mistake here. When you are finally faced with the facts and you see it really is your son, you find yourself trying to find ways to soften the impact on the rest of the family … but also it is finding a way to better absorb it for yourself.*

Extreme feelings of anger, guilt and remorse are not uncommon as parents try to find a way to live with the cause of death. Two bereaved mothers shared the following thoughts:

> *You are angry at yourself for not being able to prevent this; you are angry at the system around you for not being able to prevent it. You are also confused because what you thought you could do to prevent it didn't work.*

The media tried to fan our sense of vengeance ... but what good would that do? For myself, I needed to step back to ask what I would get out of it. So yes, I was very angry. We are looking for solace, for a way to appease the pain ... we continue to live, and there will never be closure. We still have to find ways of living with our son's death, but vengeance won't help. (Silverman 2000, p. 140)

Suicide

After a child's suicide, parents may face both the loss and an additional sense of responsibility (Shneidman & Mandelkorn 1994, Shneidman 1996). If parents feel in hindsight that they had been aware of their child's intentions, or that their efforts were inadequate to alter the outcome, then guilt and remorse may become a significant part of grieving. Some family members experience a sense of isolation and stigma as Iris Bolton (1986, p. 204) described:

I felt embarrassment. I asked myself, 'What must my friends think of me and our family? How can I ever face them again? I am so humiliated.'

And later:

I felt isolated even though people were all about. It was so easy to say 'Nobody loved him the way I did'. No one even understands my pain or can empathise with it. Worst of all, nobody wants to talk to me about what happened. Everyone avoids the subject.

Guilt may make it harder for parents to share with others, preventing them from seeking outside help. Equally, the social stigma associated with suicide may limit the support offered by family and friends (Stillion 1996). The tensions caused by violent death can be so great for the parents that surviving children, who may be experiencing similar feelings, are excluded (Rosenblatt 2000).

RECONSTRUCTING THE DYING AND THE DEATH

Many parents have a need to reconstruct mentally the circumstances of their child's death. This includes both parents who witnessed the death when events were too traumatic or confusing to have a clear picture of the tragedy and parents who were not present at the time of death. Insufficient information can lead to uncertainty, as one parent explained (Rosenblatt 2000, p. 54). '*I still have questions as to really how it happened. Why [my brother-in-law] didn't see [the car that crashed into theirs] and [our son] said they were arguing and, like I say, I don't know how much stock you can really put into what a 3 year old remembers. I still deal with that ... I wish I really knew what happened.*'

Reconstruction may be helped by postmortem information, which may give a story about the death. Knowing who, or what, was responsible for the death in situations such as murder, vehicle crash or disasters can be very important, as a mother explained (Rosenblatt 2000, p. 55).

*[The doctor went over the autopsy information with us] I think more than **anybody** else, even more than each other, reassured us that we had done nothing*

*wrong. We knew that, but it was like **he** gave us the permission to feel strong enough about that, … to feel that we had done nothing wrong and we'd done everything right. And that it was out of our control.*

Understanding the cause of death can be part of affirming the reality of the death. Funerals, too, are a way of making the death real.

FUNERALS

Funerals are a ritual that can assist to maintain the reality of the death and, as we noted in Chapter 2, can be part of the transition towards a life without the child. Iris Bolton (1986, p. 210) wrote:

It served as a ritual through which our feelings could be vented and acted out when it was too difficult to talk about them. The funeral served to affirm basic assumptions about life that were shattered by our son's death. We had to look at the meaning and purpose of life and death. The ceremony also helped us to face the truth about his death and gave us an opportunity to say goodbye.

A child's funeral is an important event for many parents and for others in the family. As Rose described (Box 3.1), it involves parents making choices about what happens to their child. Funeral choices may be limited by the nature of the death. For example, parents who have experienced an early miscarriage may decide not to have a funeral and choose to create their own special farewell ritual. Rosenblatt (2000) noted that many parents found it touching and important that many people attended the funeral. It conveyed to them that people supported them and cared about the child. One father made the following comment (Rosenblatt 2000, p. 70):

You find out who your friends are … There was over 300 people, and the guy said that he's never seen that many people for a 10-week-old baby that a lot of them didn't even get a chance to see, so it makes you feel like you got a lot of friends, a lot of people that care about you.

Dent (2000) found that all 67 parents in her study felt satisfied with their child's funeral service.

It was done as we wanted. It was very beautiful. We had 'Knocking on Heaven's Door' as the coffin went into the cremation place. A friend sang 'Amazing Grace'. My father conducted the service.

The service was lovely but very upsetting and stressful.

However, plans can go awry. Parents may be left caring and advocating for their child up until the point of cremation, as Pip described:

We got down to the place where you get people cremated, and they have that little curtain where the coffins go behind the curtain. I said to the undertaker: 'What happens to her now?' He said 'Oh, we are going to cremate her in the morning'. I said 'If you do that, I'm taking her home. I'm not leaving her with strangers overnight.' In the end the guy said 'We can do it this afternoon'.

Equally, as Rose described, funerals may appear to have been an 'incomplete' farewell to the child if there are any subsequent concerns about organ retention. This issue has arisen in the last few years in a range of countries and has caused considerable distress to parents and families.

The funeral may mark the end of a busy time when arrangements may have taken up much of the parents' time. It is often at this time point that friends and others fade away so that parents are left alone to find a way to grieve the loss of their child. In the days and weeks after the death, parents may experience a range of feelings.

PARENTS' FEELINGS AND COPING

NUMBNESS AND SHOCK

Not surprisingly, the first reaction to the death may be a resistance to acknowledge the awful truth, which parents will experience emotionally, physically and cognitively. As Sarnoff Schiff (1977, p. 24), a bereaved mother, explained, the shock or numbness may last for several weeks.

> *The numbness stayed with me for days and would come in waves just as my weeping and sorrow would come in waves. For that, a grieving parent can be thankful. If we had to face the enormity of our loss for every waking minute, I am certain it would completely envelop us and consume us and prevent us from ever again becoming whole.*

Shock may also preclude gaining or understanding information, as one father described: '*Because one is in such a state of shock, you tend not to ask the relevant questions. If you don't ask, you don't get told. People are afraid of upsetting you further.*'

ANGER

Anger may be part of grief. Iris Bolton (1986, p. 205) wrote: '*I'm losing control of myself. If I ever let myself express my guilt and anger, I'll explode all over the place. All I can do is stuff it down inside and pretend.*' Dent (2000) found that parents' anger was usually directed at others. For instance, three couples reported that the police should have been more sympathetic and less accusing when arriving on the scene after their babies had died at home. Others were angry that hospital staff had not given them sufficient information about the death, available choices (e.g. washing or dressing their dead child) and practicalities (e.g. arranging the funeral or registering the death). When cancelling state-funded child benefit and dealing with child benefit personnel, some parents, like this father, felt quite angry. '*They seemed cold and purely financially orientated. Like: "Sorry your child has died – your money has been cut to ..." (like you are in a competition). More kids, more money – never mind, try again and we can put your money up.'*

Unfortunately, in today's world, the press may play a large part in families' experiences. The sudden death of a child is newsworthy material for television and local newspapers. Contact with the media caused great anger to a third of parents (n = 67) in Dent's study (2000). Two parents described their distress: *'Totally horrifying! It was one of the most distressing parts of the tragedy'* and *'Very, very upsetting. The press phoned many times the day after the death. When reported in the papers, local and national, all of it was made up.'*

However, occasionally, the press may help. For instance, a local newspaper assisted in the installation of street-lighting in an area where a child had died.

Contact with the coroner and receiving postmortem reports also caused anger to some parents. Over a quarter of parents did not understand the answers to their questions about the results of their child's postmortem, and a minority were not allowed to ask questions. Rosenblatt (2000) found that parents also feel angry with God, or some higher being, who had allowed their child to die. They had believed God to be just, wise, caring and compassionate and all-powerful. How could such a God allow their child to die?

GUILT

When a child dies, unless room is allowed for logic, anything can serve as a starting point from which to blame oneself for the death. And where is the logic in the death of a child? Many parents find themselves searching for what they did to cause the death. As Rosenblatt (2000, p. 88) noted, *'Many parent narratives speak of feelings of guilt'*. Different sources of guilt can include surviving, activities that might have caused the death or caused God to take the child, being less than an ideal parent, not being sufficiently loving towards the child or having been absent when the child died. As Rose described, it has taken her 8 years to feel that she did all that she could have done at the time of Ruby's death.

COPING

Feelings are part of a reaction to loss. Memories, telling stories and thinking about the child can form part of loss-oriented coping. As we discussed in Chapter 3, Stroebe and Schut (2001) proposed that people move between loss- and restoration-oriented coping. The latter involves dealing with the new reality and undertaking everyday activities required of changed family roles. Bereaved parents move between a range of coping activities that include seeking information, allowing oneself to be supported by others, taking direct action, retreating into or trying to control feelings and finding ways of constructing a relationship with the deceased. Rose described her experience in the first few weeks after Ruby died. *'Sometimes I kept really busy, doing things around the house. Then at other times I would ring Mum and talk about how I felt. I went quite a bit to Ruby's grave and that helps, just to spend time thinking about her. Then it was back to cook tea and get the girls to bed.'*

THE PAIN AND DEPTH OF GRIEF

Intense feelings and associated changes in behaviour and physical health can mean that the pain and depth of parental grief is unimaginable. Three mothers described the intensity of pain, which can be both physical and emotional.

*I wanted to collapse. I wanted to die. I wanted my baby back. **I wanted my baby** back. My arms felt so empty. Where had he gone? We have been robbed of our child just as cruelly as if someone had stolen into our house in the middle of the night and murdered him.* (Diamond 1995, p. 93)

I feel very much like a time bomb and cry so much when alone, but seem like a happy lady when present with others. Really my heart aches and I am desperately unhappy. I often think when these people say: 'You are coping well', spend 5 minutes in my broken body and tell me I'm coping. They know nothing.

*You get beyond, it's so **deep within**. I mean it's such a, well words never can explain, but it's so deep. And that heaviness is so deep that that's almost far more difficult than crying ... a sexual relationship is very deep but grieving is deeper than that. Deep, deep, deep ... you find out that you have roots that you never thought you had, and you go to these roots.* (Rosenblatt 2000, p. 76)

A father described his constant pain:

The pain will never go away. We love our son so much. He was so bright. He used to help me with my spelling as it's so bad.

Each comment is different but in each there is a profound message that the death of their child has shaken them to the core. Many parents report feelings of '*going through the motions*', reflecting a sense of being detached from the situation, the outside world and themselves (Hogan, Morse & Tason 1996). Amidst the pain is also an *An intimate loneliness*, as Riches and Dawson (2000) entitled their book. It reflects an experience that is unique and isolating, even when other family members share the event. While recognising differences between individuals, it is useful to consider broad differences between mothers and fathers (see discussion on gender, p. 35), since each can influence the others' experience. The uniqueness of grieving may mean that different ways of coping emerge within the relationship.

DIFFERENCES IN MOTHERS' AND FATHERS' GRIEF

We have emphasised throughout this text, that individuals do not grieve in isolation. They grieve within a social context of which a central part may be their family. This means that a bereaved parent, with no previous experience of family death, may look to their partner as a reference point for their grief, only to find that as individuals they grieve differently (Sarnoff Schiff 1977).

FATHERS

In the time soon after death, many fathers are more likely to put their energies into practical issues, supporting their partners, controlling their emotions, rationalising the death and finding ways to divert their grief into practical activities (Hazzard, Weston & Gutteres 1992, Gilbert 1996, Moriarty, Carroll & Cotroneo 1996, McGreal, Evans & Burrow 1997). Two fathers explained their discomfort about talking of their child's death:

> I am always embarrassed that I will cry, which makes me angry. This makes me feel very low. It's as if I locked away the feelings in hospital when my son died, but the feelings have a real good pick at the locks sometimes.

> I find it hard to come to terms with my daughter's death. Sometimes I can't talk to anyone. I try not to bring it into conversation. When my partner talks about it, I find it hard to talk back to her and try to avoid it by going out.

Some fathers may prefer to release their pain in private. One father said in response to his wife's comment that he had hardly cried at all: 'That's all you know. We've this shed at work and there would be times I would lock myself in and just roar' (Riches & Dawson 1996, p. 149).

MOTHERS

Conversely, many mothers have a greater need or willingness to recognise, label, express and disclose feelings (Schwab 1992, Duncombe & Marsden 1995, Gilbert 1996). Riches and Dawson (2000) found that some mothers described losing a central part of themselves after the death, with all else becoming unimportant. Many mothers appeared to grieve more intensely, be more immersed in their grief and to feel cheated, guilty, irritable and preoccupied with thoughts of the dead child. As one mother said (Riches & Dawson 2000, p. 12), 'Nothing made sense anymore. I couldn't stand my husband near me. I went through the motions with the other children. I just felt I wasn't there.'

PARENTS TOGETHER AND SEPARATELY

Because of these different ways of grieving, couples may have difficulty in maintaining any closeness or understanding of each other's grief. This may lead to further tensions in an already stressful situation. In Rosenblatt's study (2000), parents talked about a pattern where one partner of the couple wanted to be more alone, to grieve privately, and not talk about certain things. The other partner wanted to be more in contact, to share grief and to be supported. A number of studies report that parents identify relationship difficulties connected to the bereavement (Cornwell, Nurcombe & Stevens 1977, Gilbert & Smart 1992, Gilbert 1996, Dent 2000). A mother described her feelings about this (Dijkstra 2002, p. 38):

> *Because of all the pain and sorrow, I have the feeling that my husband is avoiding me. He avoids problems, can't cope with emotions. He gets angry when I am crying, because he thinks I have to accept the situation. I suffer health problems, the consequence of stress. We find it very difficult, this should not be happening to us. I feel desperate and helpless. Every day is a struggle to survive.*

Other parents may strengthen the bond between them because they deal with their grief similarly and can support each other. The hopes and ambitions that each parent invested in their deceased child are unlikely to have been the same or to have carried the same significance. Regrets, guilt, unfinished business, special memories and specific problems associated with the lost relationship are not necessarily shared or understood by both parents (Riches & Dawson 2000). Where there are step-parents, or where partners come from different cultural and ethnic backgrounds, tensions and misunderstanding can increase (Peppers & Knapp 1980, Corwin 1995). For example, a mother's grief following the death of her son may be difficult for a new partner to understand especially if he has only just assumed the role of step-father and does not have any children of his own.

As parents grieve, many feelings are experienced and changes take place at many levels (Silverman 2000). The relationship between the parents will change frequently over the years as they deal with the death. It is not just a question of dealing with it once and for all; challenges may continue to emerge. A bereaved mother and father described their experience (Silverman 2000, p. 138):

> *I think that the reason that our marriage lasted and got better after his death was because we were pretty much in agreement even though our styles are so different. We were basically able to talk about most things and were able to live with each other's differences.*

The examples in this section indicate that, for many, the relationship between parents may provide both support and a source of tension. But what are the effects of other relationships with the family? How do parents cope with surviving children?

SUPPORT

PARENTS' EXPERIENCE OF SUPPORTING SURVIVING SIBLINGS

Sarnoff Schiff (1977, pp. 83–84), herself a bereaved mother, suggested that one of the most difficult challenges is to continue to be a parent to surviving children:

> *It means groping to find the right words and attitudes to comfort a living brother or sister ... helping to fill the void left by the dead child who formerly shared a*

table, games, a bedroom, the same preference in television. And the emptiness of not having that person to share can be unfathomable… Parenthood now becomes walking and talking and listening and hearing someone else at a time when it takes everything just to think or function for oneself.

Telling children of the death can be a hard thing to do. Sarnoff Schiff (1977, p. 93) described how she told her 4-year-old daughter:

I began by simply saying that Robby was dead. She asked, 'For how long will he be dead?' I replied, 'Forever. He will never be back'. But a 4-year old, no matter how astute, just cannot grasp 'forever'. I could see how puzzled and frightened she was.

Many parents have found that dealing with their own emotions and sharing them with their children may be difficult. Some parents find discipline difficult. One mother explained (Silverman 2000, p. 143):

It didn't work trying to be angry when he did something that he knew wasn't right.… What worked was understanding and hugging and letting him be a kid. Sometimes I had to put my foot down;… it was very difficult to sort out what is part of death and what was related to other things.

Rosenblatt (2000) found that some parents told stories of increased distancing from their surviving children for reasons such as being preoccupied or demoralised by the death and wanting to protect the children from their own grief. As one parent explained (Rosenblatt 2000, p. 157), '*I don't think [our children] ever really saw us cry.… We tried to protect them from emotion… by not showing enough of it. I don't know that they know how hurt we've been…, but then they don't tell us, "cause they probably didn't want to".*' The effect of a sudden, unexpected family death means that siblings are bereaved and are living amidst the grief of their parents. This may lead to changes such as altered behaviour. In two studies (Dent et al 1996, Dent 2000), parents reported that the changes most frequently experienced by their 150 surviving children were aggression and withdrawal. In addition, bullying, telling fibs and bedwetting were common. The majority of parents wanted more guidance and information on how to cope with these changes. Parents may struggle to know how to support their children, as Rose described in Box 3.1, and may value support from other family members. One parent commented about bereaved siblings (Hitcham 1995, p. 25):

I still can't get over how as parents you just expect them to cope and unwittingly give them the message not to intrude and just to get on with their own lives. If only I could have my time again, I'd explain much more right from the beginning bringing it into normal everyday conversation.

PARENTS' EXPERIENCE OF SOCIAL SUPPORT

In Chapter 1, we emphasised the social and cultural contexts within which individuals grieve. The current cultural environment means that child deaths are less common in Western society than in past times. Customs and attitudes, appropriate in a society characterised by a high childhood mortality rate, which provided support and comfort for those involved have disappeared almost completely as the frequency of such deaths has fallen to low levels (Mulkay 1993). This influences the resources and support that are available to bereaved parents. Parents' social context includes the family setting with other bereaved family members and the extrafamilial setting of friends, colleagues, neighbours, acquaintances, other bereaved families and health professionals. Other people provide resources in the form of social support (Cohen & Syme 1985), which may be emotional, informational or instrumental (practical) help (Thuen 1997). Lehman, Ellard and Wortman (1986) found that while would-be supporters knew what kind of behaviours and patterns of communication would be helpful to the bereaved, they were unable to offer such help. This, they suggested, arises from uncertainty and from lack of experience, causing people to fall back on responses, such as, 'You will soon get over it'. Discomfort on the part of the other person may lead to avoidance of the bereaved parent. One mother described her anger and frustration at such practices:

> The attitude of mothers/parents frustrated and upset me to such an extent that I repeatedly questioned my own sanity. I wanted to scream at them 'It isn't catching if you speak to me – it won't cause it to happen to you.' Even close friends find it a difficult subject so avoid it (and you). The longer the words are put off, the harder it becomes until eventually it is easier not to speak at all.

In contrast, when there is acknowledgement of the loss, such as receiving letters of condolence, this is appreciated by many parents.

> I didn't want sympathy or religious clichés. The letters that I found most comforting were those that showed me how much **they** missed her – how deeply they were grieving as well as me. I knew she was special, but wanted everyone else to know it too. (Riches & Dawson 2000, p. 159)

> And even people sending cards. … We really look forward to getting mail 'cause we'd get cards. (Rosenblatt 2000, p. 164)

Riches and Dawson's work (2000) found that many parents felt that their bereavement identified their true friends. Some found that one special person was willing to listen to their story repeatedly and was able 'to gently nudge their friend into noticing the effects of their difficult behaviour on other family members' (Riches & Dawson 2000, p. 155). Many parents speak about the importance of having listeners. These may be friends or, as Rose described, other parents at a mutual help group such as the Baby Bereavement Group. Many parents describe the value of support from other family members, who are also bereaved by the death of the child. Anne Diamond (1995, p. 94) wrote: 'My mother arrived. We fell into each other's arms. I could feel the double burden of grief in her embrace. She was breaking her heart for Supi, but also for me. She looked so terribly betrayed by what had happened.' Similarly, Rose described the support that her mother gave her:

> I ring Mum every day – that's the way we are. I mean I can just ring up Mum when I feel sad and when I feel happy and when we talk I know she remembers

all the days that are hard for me. … And she keeps my feet on the ground. When I moan about the girls she says to me, 'you've got to be a bit more understanding' because sometimes I forget how deeply they've been affected by it.

Sometimes, other family members may not appreciate the parents' loss, because it has little meaning for them. One mother described her experience having had a miscarriage (Moulder 2001, p. 105): '*It's a horrible, lonely, experience. My sister's baby died the same month and she got all the family sympathy because we all knew the baby – it was real to all of us. My baby was real to me and my partner.*' Finally, as Silverman (2000) suggested, even if support is available, not everyone is receptive to it. Some families invite others into their lives, while others want to do as much as they can for themselves. Therefore, what help is provided, and by whom, has to be respectful and suited to the family (Silverman 2000).

PARENTS' EXPERIENCE OF PROFESSIONAL SUPPORT

Dent's study (2000) focused on bereaved parents' perception of support in hospital and community. The majority of parents reported that hospital care at the time of death had generally been 'good', although some would have liked more choices and information. However, follow-up care in the community was greatly lacking, leaving the majority of parents feeling very isolated and alone. Of the parents who responded, 13% had received on-going bereavement support from their GP and 12% from their health visitor. Some parents made the following comments:

Professionals should get more involved. They should contact the parents afterwards. We could have gone off our heads here and no-one would have known. They should check parents are handling it OK.

The past months have been difficult. I row with my partner and have run out of comforting words when she wakes crying. The only support we have had has been from a few friends and colleagues, although the GP has seen my wife on several occasions.

I feel there is a need for someone in the local authority who could contact families soon after the death to talk about many questions.

My partner visited his GP to ask for help of a psychologist, but he was given a bottle of pills which just zonked him right out. My partner is very depressed at the moment and I feel it has all been left to me to handle.

When asked what advice parents would give to health professionals, the following comments were forthcoming:

Always have time to listen. More support at home by the health visitor is needed, not just at the time but afterwards.

They should stop telling people it will get better in time. You don't get over the death of your child in a few months.

Never be afraid to show you care. The death of a child is extremely distressing. Be honest and grieve with the parents.

My husband had little or no support. Everyone seemed to bother about me and not him.

Dent (2000) found that parents did not expect to have to ask for help from professionals; they felt it should have been forthcoming since they were the ones who had been affected. When they had known the GP or health visitor prior to the death, the parents felt let down when the health professionals did not visit. Even when a letter was put through their door from their health visitor, asking them to ring if they wanted anything, they were uncertain as to what help could be offered, since 'health visitors deal with live babies' and their child was no longer alive. Moulder (2001) identified that mothers experienced similar issues after miscarriage. Provision of support by health professionals is discussed further in Chapters 6–8. So, with or without the assistance of social resources, how do parents find different ways to live with their loss and adjust to a changed world?

FINDING WAYS TO LIVE WITH A CHILD'S DEATH

In 'Setting the scene', we discussed the different ways that parents find to live with the death of their child. This includes different relationships with the child (McClowry et al 1987) and different roles that the child may hold in their lives (Marwit & Klass 1995). We also explored the idea of personal resources for grieving (Riches & Dawson 2000). These include beliefs, previous experiences, knowledge and social support that individuals use to make sense of their experience. Rituals, memories, tokens of remembrance, telling stories and thinking about the child may help to confirm the death and assist relearning and adjusting to a changed world.

Many parents are worried that they may forget their child (Malkinson & Bar-Tur 1999). Memories and tokens of remembrance emphasise connections between child and parent (Klass 1996) and can remind parents of their own worth, and that of their child. Parents may use tokens of remembrance such as photographs or clothing as a trigger to share stories of the dead child with family members and other people (Riches & Dawson 1998). When other people do not share or listen to the memories, parents may feel upset or let down. Pip described (p. 104) wanting grandparents to remember her daughter Gracie. Some parents become extremely protective of memorabilia. For instance, they may not want other children to play with the deceased child's toys or they may want to keep a child's room as it was before the death (Edelstein 1984). A bereaved mother described the physical place where her daughter Leanne's belongings were kept (Rosenblatt 2000, p. 129). '*As you can see, her pictures are up. The albums down there are all Leanne's. … Her clothes are still here. Her animals are still here. And Leanne's room is there. You can walk in, see her Barbie dolls, see her animals. The nieces and nephews … know that … you have to have permission to play with Leanne's stuff.*'

Many parents speak about tokens of remembrance that remind them of their child (Rosenblatt 2000, p. 198). *'Everywhere you look there's something. That was something on the refrigerator there that she did. She made it ... always making ... sketches and ... little things that probably, at the time, didn't mean anything.'* Some parents plant a tree as a living reminder of their child. Remembering birthdays or lighting candles on special days are personal rituals that may be important to keep their child's memory alive. Other parents have images that retain a continuing place for the child in the family, as a mother described (Rosenblatt 2000, p. 133): *'When I picture my kids, I picture all five of them ... but the ones who died are still babies ... I take a deep breath, but I always think of five. So I guess in that sense they are always with me. It's not like I had one and then a space and then two, three. It's one, two, three, four, five.'*

Some parents feel that others want them to 'get over' the death like a person recovers from a cold (Rosenblatt 2000). Such a phrase can be interpreted to mean having no feelings of grief and even forgetting their child. This may not feel useful or reasonable to parents. Two mothers constructed their view of bereavement in the following descriptions:

> *You live everything by firsts, you know. Like the first week you go 'Gee, last Tuesday I was doing this and this with [the baby] ... Well, this is only a week ago, and he's not here any more. Well, how weird!' You know and it was really tough, and then you go to the first month. You know, and then you go to anniversaries, birthdays ... like all those firsts. You remember to the day.* (Martin 1998, pp. 97–98)

> *We know now that we cannot control what happens to us, but we can take charge of how we respond. We can choose to survive or we can choose to be devastated. I can no longer change the destiny of my loved one, but I can be sure that my life will be more meaningful as a result of this experience. I can survive.* (Bolton 1986, p. 211)

Many researchers have found that grief for the death of a child may continue for a long time, even a lifetime (Rosen 1986, Rubin 1993, 1996, Lang, Gottlieb & Amsel 1996, Malkinson & Bar-Tur 1999). The sudden death of a child has the potential to shatter lives and requires people to find a way to reconstruct a view of the world that they can live with. As Rose described in her story (Box 3.1), this may take years of intense and prolonged thought and activity. It may include telling and retelling the story of their child's death to find a way to adjust to the changed reality. Making meaning may also involve exploring questions such as 'What is the meaning of life?' Some parents, like Rose, find a meaning or a purpose for the death. One mother explained a new insight, gained 2 years after her daughter died:

> *One of the best and most useful things I have read is 'out of adversity comes a seed of equal or greater benefit'. This is a great philosophy for life. I don't know how I would advise anyone unfortunate enough to go through this, as I know it can tear your life down and turn you into a miserable, over-protective wretch. Or by your own decision, you can accept it, learn from it and move on.*

Sometimes experiences of loss can enable personal growth that is cognitive, emotional, spiritual and social. Two parents described their perspective of living with the loss:

> *Gradually our guilt turned to regret, as we continued to share and talk. Our strength returned, bearing the gifts of laughter without guilt, of joy, of faith in God, and of confidence in the future.* (Bolton 1986, p. 210)

> *My dear son's death had a tremendous impact on me, but it has been an impetus for positive change and growth in me. I had him for a few short years, but he has given a special love to my life. He can't receive my love, but I can send it to him by giving to others.*

There are some parents who do not find ways to live purposefully and constructively with their child's death. Perspectives of such a place have been described as complicated grief (Rando 1993) and difficult deaths (Riches & Dawson 2000). This is discussed further in Chapter 8. Finally, for some parents, deciding to have another child may be part of living with the death of a child. As Rose described in her story, such decisions are not easy. They may lead to revisiting the place of the dead child in the family, revisiting the meaning of their death and finding new ways to move on as a family with a new member.

SUMMARY

Many of the words in this chapter have come from bereaved parents; it is clear that their grief is deep, intense individual and long lasting. Supporting those who are bereaved requires an awareness of the uniqueness of each individual's response.

SUMMARY POINTS

- Parents experience a range of feelings such as shock, numbness, guilt, resentment and anger, which may be accompanied by changes in behaviour and physical well-being.
- The funeral is an important event, which may bring comfort and solace to some parents, especially when it is well attended and others remember the dead child positively.
- Differences in grieving may bring added tensions to a couple's relationship.
- Many parents are aware of their surviving children's grief but may be unsure how to help them and would appreciate guidance and information.
- Parents have different ways of living with the death, making meaning of their experience and constructing a relationship with their dead child.

REFERENCES

Bolton I 1986 Death of a child by suicide. In: Rando TA (ed) Parental loss of a child. Research Press, Champaign, IL, p 201–212

Brice CW 1991a Paradoxes of maternal mourning. Psychiatry 54: 1–12

Brice CW 1991b What forever means: an empirical existential–phenomenological investigation of maternal mourning. Journal of Phenomenological Psychology 22: 16–38

Cohen S, Syme SL 1985 Issues in the study of social support. In: Cohen S, Syme SL (eds) Social support and health. Academic Press, New York

Cornwell J, Nurcombe B, Stevens L 1977 Family response to loss of a child by sudden infant death syndrome. Medical Journal of Australia 1: 656–658

Corwin MD 1995 Cultural issues in bereavement therapy: the social construction of mourning. In Session: Psychotherapy in Practice, 1: 23–41

Dent A 2000 Support for families whose child dies suddenly from accident or illness. PhD thesis, School of Policy Studies, University of Bristol, UK

Dent A, Condon L, Fleming P et al 1996 A study of bereavement care after sudden and unexpected death. Archives of Disease in Childhood 74: 522–526

Diamond A 1995 A gift from Sebastian. A story of a cot death. Boxtree, London

Dijkstra I 2002 The aftermath of losing a child. Bereavement Care 21: 38–40

Duncombe J, Marsden D 1995 Workaholics and whinging women: theorising intimacy and emotion work – the last frontier of gender inequality? Sociological Review 43: 150–170

Edelstein L 1984 Maternal bereavement: coping with the unexpected death of a child. Praeger, New York

Finlay I, Dallimore D 1991 Your child is dead. British Medical Journal 302: 1524–1525

Gatenby B 1998 For the rest of our lives after the death of a child. Reed Books, Auckland, NZ

Gilbert KR 1996 'We've had the same loss, why don't we have the same grief?' Loss and differential grief in families. Death Studies 20: 269–283

Gilbert KR, Smart LS 1992 Coping with infant or fetal loss: the couple's healing process. Brunner, New York

Hazzard A, Weston J, Gutteres C 1992 After a child's death: factors related to parental bereavement. Journal of Development and Behavioural Paediatrics 13: 24–30

Hitcham M 1995 Direct work techniques with the siblings of children dying from cancer. In: Smith S, Pennells M (eds) Interventions with bereaved children. Jessica Kingsley, London, p 24–44

Hogan N, Morse JM, Tason M 1996 Toward an experiential theory of bereavement. OMEGA, Journal of Death and Dying 33: 43–65

Klass D 1996 The deceased child in the psychic and social worlds of bereaved parents during the resolution of grief. In: Klass D, Silverman P, Nickman S (eds) Continuing bonds. New understandings of grief. Taylor & Francis, Washington, DC, p 199–215

Lang A, Gottlieb LN, Amsel R 1996 Predictors of husbands' and wives' grief reactions following infant death: the role of marital intimacy. Death Studies 20: 33–57

Lehman DR, Ellard JH, Wortman CB 1986 Social support the bereaved: recipients' and providers' perspectives on what is helpful. Journal of Consulting and Clinical Psychology 52: 218–231

Lehman DR, Lang EL, Wortman CB et al 1989 Long term effects of sudden bereavement: marital and parent–child relationships and children's reactions. Journal of Family Psychology 2: 344–367

Malkinson R, Bar-Tur L 1999 The ageing of grief in Israel: a perspective of bereaved parents. Death Studies 23: 413–431

Mander R, 1994 Loss and bereavement in childbearing. Blackwell Scientific, Oxford

Martin K 1998 When a baby dies of SIDS: the parents' grief and search for reason. Qual Institute Press, University of Alberta, Edmonton, Alberta

Marwit SJ Klass D 1995 Grief and the role of the inner representation of the deceased. OMEGA, Journal of Death and Dying 30: 283–298

McClowry S, Davies E, May K et al 1987 The empty space phenomenon. Death Studies 11: 361–374

McGreal D, Evans BJ Burrows GD 1997 Gender differences in coping following loss of a child through miscarriage or stillbirth: a pilot study. Stress Medicine 13: 159–165

Moriarty HJ, Carroll R, Cotroneo M 1996 Differences in bereavement reactions with couples following the death of a child. Research in Nursing and Health 19: 61–69

Moulder C 2001 Miscarriage: women's experiences and needs, 2nd edn. Routledge, London

Mulkay M 1993 Social death in Britain. In: Clark D (ed) The sociology of death. Blackwell, Oxford

Peppers LG, Knapp RJ 1980 Motherhood and mourning. Perinatal death. Praeger, New York

Rando T 1986 The unique issues and impact of the death of a child. In: Rando T (ed) Parental loss of a child. Research Press, Champaign IL, p 3–44

Rando T 1993 Treatment of complicated mourning. Research Press, Champaign, IL

Redmond L 1996 Sudden violent death. In: Doka K (ed) Living with grief after sudden loss. Taylor & Francis, Philadelphia, PA, p 53–73

Riches G, Dawson P 1996 Communities of feeling: the culture of bereaved families. Mortality 1: 143–161

Riches G, Dawson P 1998 Lost children, living memories: the role of photographs in processes of grief and adjustment among bereaved parents. Death Studies 22: 121–140

Riches G, Dawson P 2000 An intimate loneliness: supporting bereaved parents and siblings. Open University Press, Buckingham, UK

Rosen H 1986 Unspoken grief: coping with childhood sibling loss. Lexington Books, Toronto

Rosenblatt P 2000 Parents' grief: narratives of loss and relationship. Brunner/Mazel, Philadelphia, PA

Rosenblatt P 2002 Guest editorial: grief in families. Mortality 7: 125–126

Rubin S 1993 The death of a child is forever: the life course impact of child loss. In: Stroebe M, Stroebe W, Hansson R (eds) Handbook of bereavement: theory, research and intervention. Cambridge University Press, New York, p 285–299

Rubin S 1996 The wounded family: bereaved parents and the impact of adult child loss. In: Klass D, Silverman P, Nickman S (eds) Continuing bonds. New understandings of grief. Taylor & Francis, Washington, DC, p 217–234

Sarnoff Schiff H 1977 The bereaved parent. Souvenir Press, London

Schwab R 1992 Effects of a child's death on the marital relationship: a preliminary study. Death Studies 16: 141–154

Shneidman E 1996 The suicidal mind. Oxford University Press, New York

Shneidman E, Mandelkorn P 1994 Some facts and fables of suicide. In: Shneidman E, Farberrow NL, Litman R (eds) The psychology of suicide: a clinician's guide to evaluation and treatment. Jason Aaronson, Northvale, NJ, p 87–95

Silverman P 2000 Never too young to know. Oxford University Press, New York

Stewart A 2000 When an infant grandchild dies: family matters. Unpublished doctoral dissertation. School of Nursing, University of Wellington, Wellington, NZ

Stillion JM 1996 Survivors of suicide. In: Doka K (ed) Living with grief and loss. Taylor & Francis, Philadelphia, PA, p 41–53

Stroebe M, Schut H 2001 Meaning making in the dual process of coping with bereavement. In: Neimeyer R (ed) Meaning reconstruction and the experience of loss. American Psychological Association, Washington, DC, p 55–75

Thuen F 1997 Social support after the loss of an infant child: a long-term perspective. Scandinavian Journal of Psychology 38: 103–110

USEFUL SOURCES FOR NURSES AND MIDWIVES

Kohner N, Henley A 2001 When a baby dies, 2nd edn. Routledge, London

Moulder C 2001 Miscarriage: women's experiences and needs, 2nd edn. Routledge, London

Riches G, Dawson P 2000 An intimate loneliness: supporting bereaved parents and siblings. Open University Press, Buckingham, UK

Rosenblatt P 2000 Parent grief: narratives of loss and relationship. Brunner/Mazel, Philadelphia, PA

Family bereavement: the experience of surviving children

The room is silent, silent and dark
Four pairs of eyes stare anxiously
As the sleeping baby gasps for breath
Then begins to breathe normally again

The sleeping baby lies soundly in his
Loving Grandfather's arms
He stirs but doesn't wake
This baby is surrounded with love
The love of his Parents and
The love of his Grandparents

This baby is also in pain and suffering
He is dying and no one can help

Not the doctors or anyone
The only help he can get is love
Love is all anyone can give him

Suddenly the baby starts gasping again
But this time he doesn't begin to breathe
Normally again
It stops ... everything is quiet
All that can be heard is the sobbing
And the question in every one's mind
Why us? Why did it have to happen to us?

The Sleeping Baby
by Rochelle the sister of Matthew

INTRODUCTION

The last chapter focused on parents' grief as experienced by them. This chapter is about the grief experience of siblings using, wherever possible, quotes from them. We have also used other material based on the limited research that is available from other situations where children are bereaved, such as following the death of a parent. It must be noted that it is generally adults, as researchers and clinicians, who describe and construct meaning about children's experiences; hence much of what is written is from an adult perspective.

In this chapter we explore children's understanding of death. While this knowledge is generally developed from studies with children who are not bereaved, it gives a base from which to understand something of children's concepts of death. We look at bereaved children's feelings, choices that are available to them and children's behaviour following a death. We conclude by considering the effect that the family may have on surviving siblings, and how they can construct an on-going relationship with the dead sibling. As one chapter on the subject is very limited, a further reading list is given at the end of the chapter.

THE FORGOTTEN MOURNERS

The poem from Rochelle was included as part of the study on grandparent bereavement (Stewart 2000) and emphasises the awareness of a young sibling aged 6 years when her brother died. Her words illustrate clearly the effect that death can have on a young child.

Bereaved brothers and sisters have been called 'the forgotten mourners' (Hindmarch 1995, p. 37). Children's reactions to the loss of a sibling, as opposed to the death of a parent, have received much less attention from researchers and writers interested in childhood bereavement (Segal et al 1995). Why should this be? It may be for a variety of reasons including:

- adult discomfort with children's concrete/bald questions
- lack of understanding that children are different and not mini-adults
- sibling relationships being considered secondary and relatively unimportant compared with parent–child relationships (Hogan & DeSantis 1992, Segal et al 1995)
- children being less able than parents to claim a voice; for example, parents' grief has been voiced over the last 20 years through mutual help groups such as The Compassionate Friends
- ethical tensions of doing research with children.

The consequence of being overlooked means that there is limited information representing bereaved siblings' experience and, although there may be common threads, we cannot generalise to all siblings on the basis of the experiences of some siblings. While an increasing number of books and articles are now being written about bereaved children, few are based on studies that give definitive information about this population. The research findings on childhood grief are often inconsistent and differ between studies. As Worden (1996) suggested, this may be for several reasons. Some studies fail to use a demographically matched non-bereaved control group. Without such controls it is difficult to ascertain whether the observed behaviour is a result of bereavement, age, gender or developmental differences. Second, lack of standardised assessment means that it is difficult to make comparisons across studies. Parents, teachers and sometimes children are asked about children's reactions and feelings; all have different perspectives. In addition, many studies use small, unrepresentative samples of bereaved children and study differing age groups. Finally, the majority of studies are cross-sectional and not longitudinal, which means the long-term effects of children's grief have not been studied in detail.

THE SIBLING RELATIONSHIP

As Bank and Kahn (1982, p. 5) noted, *'We had been taught that siblings are, at best, minor actors on the stage of human development, and their influence is supposed to be fleeting, and that it is the parents who principally determine one's identity. The prevailing theories of human development seem strangely silent about siblings.'* The fact that the sibling relationship is unique and likely to be the longest social connection an individual will ever experience is often overlooked (Rando 1989). Attachments between siblings shape their personality and sense of place in the world as much as attachments to parents. Siblings share a range of experiences and activities; they may confide in each other or challenge parental authority (Martinson & Campos 1991). Nonetheless, each has a unique experience in the family, dependent on age, birth order and the relationships between parents and other siblings (Dunn & Plomin 1990). The death of a brother or sister has consequences for self-identity, relationships with parents and other surviving siblings as well as for long-term relationships in adult life (Lewis & Schonfield 1994, Robinson & Mahon 1997).

WHAT AND HOW DO CHILDREN UNDERSTAND ABOUT DEATH?

So when a brother or sister dies, what understanding do children have of the death? This section has been included because health professionals attending the workshops we run often ask for details of children's grief at different ages. However, it must be stressed that age is only **one** factor in understanding children's concepts of death. While age gives a useful guideline, it is no substitute for really hearing what any individual child has to say. Because of the diversity, this is the only sure way of understanding an individual child's comprehension, fears and anxieties arising from the death.

A mature view of death has been described as one in which there is a comprehension of the universality, irreversibility, non-functioning and causality of death (Speece 1984, Wass 1984, Brent et al 1996). Causality refers to the understanding of why people die and implies more than that the person had an illness or was in an accident. It encompasses the understanding that everyone dies, so that with life comes death (Silverman 2000).

Research with children has primarily explored how children spontaneously characterise death in their comments, stories, play and drawings (Nagy 1948, Lonetto 1980). It has included what children understand about the implications of death to their physical selves: such as what happens after death, what changes with death, what or who can die (Kenyon 2001). Emphasis has been on how similar children's concepts are to those of adults, that is, the maturity of their concepts of death (Kenyon 2001). However, it would appear that cognitive ability, age and past death experiences all play a part in children's understanding. Much of the research on children's understanding of death has focused on non-bereaved children and needs to be understood in that context.

COGNITIVE ABILITY

In a recent paper, Kenyon (2001) found that studies of cognitive ability continue to yield inconclusive results about children's comprehension of death. Intelligence appears to be related to awareness of death concepts, and in particular verbal ability, which is related to the understanding of universality, irreversibility and non-functioning. Therefore, verbal ability might contribute to a child's understanding of, and communication about, components that require abstract reasoning such as universality and non-functioning. However, as Kenyon (2001) indicated, age continues to be the only strong predictor of all components, although, as with cognitive ability, there have been differing findings.

AGE OF UNDERSTANDING DEATH

In Kenyon's review of research into children's conceptions of death (2001), she concluded by suggesting that children understand death as a changed state by about 3 years of age. By around 5 or 6 years, they understand that death is universal, but understanding of what causes death comes slightly later. In general, Kenyon noted that current measures do not detect a complete understanding of universality, irreversibility, non-functioning and personal mortality until about 10 years. However, children's conceptions of death are multi-faceted and affected by factors including:

- verbal ability to communicate
- personal experience
- families' cultural and religious beliefs
- emotional factors especially anxiety and fear of death.

Silverman (2000) has noted that bereaved children's understanding of death does not break down into clear age-specific categories. Their understanding is not just a cognitive exercise in what they think about death (Bluebond-Langner 1996). Children deal with the impact of death at personal, social and emotional levels; consequently, their cognitive understanding may be inconsistent with their level of maturity and may differ from those children who have not experienced death.

From 0 to 2 years

Children under the age of 2 years will have little understanding of the concept of death (Dyregrov 1991, Rathbone 1996, Silverman 2000). However, when their main carer is affected by a stressful situation, they may react by erratic eating and crying patterns and feeling irritable (Rathbone 1996). Toddlerhood means that language and mobility are developing as well as a sense that people and things continue to exist outside their view (Silverman 2000). Toddlers have little understanding of how death differs from going away.

From 2 to 5 years

Children aged 2 to 5 years are able to use the word 'death' without understanding the full meaning. Because they may see death as reversible, they may not grasp that all the functions of life have ceased (Dyregrov 1991). This may lead to questions such as: *'When will my baby sister come back?' 'Who will give the baby milk up in heaven'* (Dyregrov 1991, p. 9). Children at this age have limited understanding of time, so to say that a death is forever will probably mean little. For this reason, children may not react to the news when told. They may need to be told the same story repeatedly until eventually the truth is absorbed. They may not have the language capacity to describe their emotions nor to ask for what they need. They are often unable to draw comfort from spoken statements in the same way that adults can.

At this age, children are very involved with the basic physical aspects of living such as eating, sleeping and excreting. They can be very curious about what will become of the dead body and may ask questions about how the dead person will eat, drink and excrete (Silverman 2000). Parents may be thrown by the blatancy of such questions at a time when they are grieving and feeling very sensitive. Silverman (2000) suggested that by the age of 4 years children have a limited and unclear understanding of the word 'death'. Many may still believe in the power of their own magical thinking and may believe that they have caused the death.

From 5 to 9 years

Older children between the ages of 5 and 9 years begin to understand that death is permanent, but they see death as happening to other people not themselves (Corr 1984). Death is usually seen in the guise of a frightening person whom they can avoid if they are careful. At this age, they may have a preoccupation with the rituals surrounding death and, if excluded from such rituals, they may imagine things far worse than the reality. Simple, honest explanations avoid ambiguity and may help them to feel more secure in a confused and unsure world. Explanations can help children to build trust in the adults who may be involved. However, the death of a sibling may raise feelings of their own mortality, giving rise to fears for their own safety. Younger children's understanding of death is often complicated by the attempts of others, especially parents, to protect them from the raw knowledge of the death. Consequently, children may struggle to reconcile their own understanding with information offered by others.

Adolescence

During the past 50 years or so, adolescence in Western societies has become progressively longer, lasting up to 10 years (Herbert & Harper-Dorton 2002). By adolescence, young people will generally know that death is universal, inevitable and irreversible. The grief for a deceased sibling is compounded by other changes. Adolescence has been described as '*a time of life when the only thing you can be sure of is that you won't be sure of anything*' (P Vine, personal communication, 1994). During teenage years, a young person has to cope with various stresses relating to body image, self-concept, relationships, peer pressure, sexual identity and parental expectations. These factors, combined with increased independence and the gradual withdrawal from parental influence, can result in a child experiencing overwhelming feelings of loss and insecurity (Hallam & Vine 1996). They may fear losing control over their emotions and may mask their reactions through their risk-taking behaviours (Dyregrov 1991). Therefore, when teenagers are bereaved, they have to cope with the death, all its complexities and a myriad of concurrent changes.

CHILDREN'S EXPERIENCE OF GRIEF

Having considered the development of understanding death, what do children experience when they lose a sibling? Here we should consider both the range of feelings and their reaction to the rituals that surround a death.

FEELINGS

In Chapter 3, parents described a range of feelings such as shock, numbness, disbelief, guilt anger, and sadness. Do bereaved children experience similar feelings? In the following quotes, a wide range of feelings are described including shock, disbelief, anger, guilt and sadness.

Shock and disbelief

Children, like adults, do not react in one way when told the news that someone has died (Dyregrov 1991). There is a wide variation in how they receive the news. The most common reactions are shock, disbelief, dismay, protest and apathy. Some children, especially younger ones, may refuse to accept the death and firmly maintain this in an effort to keep the painful fact at a distance (Dyregrov 1991). Very often such children will continue with usual activities. The following quotes describe some of the feelings of siblings:

> I just couldn't believe it. He told my mother, made sure she called another adult to be with her, and left. I needed to hear it myself. I wanted him to say it wasn't true. Of course he couldn't. (Jocelyn aged 17; Silverman 2000, p. 153)

> The shock I faced was the death of my brother just a few short weeks ago. I have never experienced this kind of shock before in my life and I never want to again. Words cannot describe the feelings I had or still have, as it changes all the time, never the same emotions. (Lisa aged 14; Barnard & Kane 1995, p. 258)

> It was almost impossible to believe that my brother chose to kill himself. I knew he was unhappy, but I couldn't imagine he would do this. My mind raced with all sorts of questions about what I could have done. I was so angry. Then I just sort of shut off. Otherwise, I don't know how I would have got through the funeral. (Sibling after his brother's suicide; Silverman 2000, p. 153)

Guilt

Altschul (1988) and Silverman (2000) have suggested that guilt is not an issue for most bereaved children, although they posit that some young children around the age of 6 or 7 years can believe they have caused the death just by thinking about it and, therefore, feel guilty when it happens. Dyregrov (1991) cited his earlier study in 1988, based on follow-up of bereaved children from all families in one region of Norway who had lost children over a 3-year period. He noted that guilt was not overtly evident. Conversely, Riches and Dawson (2000) believed that feelings of guilt appear to be a recurring characteristic of sibling grief:

> I felt sad in my heart. Fear was a lump in my throat.
> In my head I felt guilty. I thought it was my fault.
> I was so angry, the anger coming out of my head, my eyes, everywhere.
> (11-year-old boy; Hitcham 1995, p. 35)

> I wonder if you'll get mad at me if I tell you this. It's been bothering me for a long time. Have you ever heard of magic wishes? Once when I was little and you were littler, I wished you'd go away for ever. I didn't like you having all the attention ... And then when you did go away forever, I knew I had magic wishes. Those kind of wishes are scary. ... But now I'm older, I know there aren't any magic wishes, so I don't feel bad about wishing you were gone. (11-year-old Alicia; Sims 1986, p. 13)

Similarly, Farrant (1998) told the story of Francesca, whose favourite sister died. She felt guilty because she was still alive, and guilty because she felt it was her fault that her sister had died. She was unable to talk of these feelings for many years. Self-reproach can result from the last meeting with the dead sibling and from not having a chance to say goodbye. As one sibling described (Dyregrov 1991, p. 22), it can include regrets and a sense of 'if only…':

> *The last thing we did was to quarrel.*
> *I so much wish I could have told him how much I loved him.*
> *I never got the chance to say a proper farewell.*

Riches and Dawson (2000) suggested that adults might dismiss children's guilt as irrational. This may be one reason that parents and others do not recognise the burden of guilt carried by children, and particularly adolescent siblings, for many years after the death.

Anger

Anger and acting out is a common reaction (Dyregrov 1991). Younger children often show their grief in a direct and open way by hitting and kicking. The anger may be directed against death for having taken the dead person, at God for letting it happen, at adults for excluding them, at others (or themselves) who might have prevented it, and even at the dead person for deserting them (Dyregrov 1991).

> *I'm mad and sad at the same time, even now sometimes. What do I do with this anger? You can't go around banging cars or people. I keep a lump in my throat… sometimes I can't even swallow it, but it comes back… two or three times a day.* (Dan aged 8; Silverman 2000, p. 157)

> *I'm so mixed up inside. I don't know what to think anymore. Sometimes I'm really mad at you. You left me! And I really wanted to be a big sister. Sometimes I'm guilty too. I wasn't with you when you left. Maybe I could have saved you.* (11-year-old Alicia; Sims 1986, p. 22)

Sadness

Sadness and longing appear in different ways. Some children cry frequently and can at times be inconsolable. Younger children have a short sadness-span and are usually not sad for long periods at a time (Dyregrov 1991).

> *Elsie (4 years) would spend long periods of time in front of her dead sister's picture. Now and then when she was sad, she cried but would not admit that it was her sister she cried for. She said it was because of things like having headaches or a pain in her leg, or that she had nothing to do.* (Dyregrov 1991, p. 18)

> *After Louise left I felt sad all over and could not stop crying because I had lost my best friend. I had no-one to play with and keep me warm. Just seeing her smile made me feel warm inside. At school I felt very sad because I missed her so.… My heart is broken and sad. I have lots of fears. Sometimes I lock myself in my bedroom. I just want to shut myself away from the world.* (10-year-old Emma; Hitcham 1995, p. 34)

At first I was shocked; that was the only feeling I can remember at the beginning. Now it is just sad and angry...angry because she had to go and sad because I loved her more than anything. (13-year-old; Silverman 2000, p. 98)

My sister got run over. A car came and ran her over. I was sad – it was my brother's fault. He pushed her on the road. (5-year-old Emma; Ward 1996, p. 139)

Rosen (1986) focused her study on 15–20 year olds who had lost a sibling in childhood. Using questionnaires as a means of data collection, she asked 159 young adults about their perceptions of how loss had affected their lives and that of their families. She found that the siblings described feelings of disbelief, numbness, guilt, sadness, loneliness, anger and confusion. Often they did not share these feelings with anyone. There was little open communication reported among family members, and there were alterations in family interactions, which caused new and dysfunctional family patterns of behaviour. Siblings reported that they frequently felt the need to comfort their parents and to make up to them for the loss.

Worden (1996) compared his study on grief following death of a parent with the work of Davies and McCown, who recorded the responses of 75 school children in 50 families following the death of a sibling during the first year of loss (McCown & Pratt 1985, McCown 1987, Davies 1987, 1988a,b, 1991). Worden concluded that the loss of a sibling does not portend more emotional/behavioural problems than the loss of a parent. Sadness, crying, anxiety, guilt, anger and acting out behaviour were present in both groups.

RITUALS SURROUNDING THE DEATH

As Rando (1986) suggested, rituals have important functions, not just for adults but for children too. They help to make the unreal 'real', counteract fantasies and allow an opportunity to say goodbye (Dyregrov 1991). Riches and Dawson (2000) found that many of the young people they worked with expressed the notion of invisibility when it came to rituals. Some research indicates that many benefit emotionally from being included at every stage. This includes seeing the body and attending the funeral and cremation (Lauer et al 1985, Hogan & DeSantis 1994). Children, like adults, generally appreciate being offered choices. McCown (1987) studied factors relating to bereaved children's behavioural adjustment. She noted that some children below the age of 5 years of age might show an increase in behavioural problems if they enter into rituals without preparation or proper support. Similarly, Silverman (2000) and Riches and Dawson (2000) have suggested that all children need preparation before being involved with rituals.

Seeing the body

Sometimes children demand to see their sibling, as Dyregrov (1991, p. 59) found:

Nine year old Susan was not at home when her parents took her sister to the hospital where she died shortly thereafter. She demanded to see her sister, because it was so strange and sad that she was suddenly gone, and that she would never see her again.

If children are excluded then regret and bitterness may follow. Dyregrov (1991, p. 60) described the following situation of George, aged 9:

[he] was very disappointed about not seeing his mother following her death. He was at the hospital where the adults go to see her but no-one offered him the opportunity to participate. His father did not have enough knowledge about his needs and did not know that children were allowed to take part on such occasions. Later Greg's father said this was something hospital personnel should have informed him of.

The funeral

A funeral is a special family occasion that marks the end of someone's life. Walter (1996, p. 14) described the funeral or memorial service as part of survivors 'writing the last chapter'. Both the funeral and practicalities leading up to it mark a turning point in facing up to the truth that a child has died (Raphael 1994). Therefore, to exclude children from either contributing to the arrangements or attending the service is to deny them an opportunity of saying goodbye and being part of a family ritual (Lauer et al 1985). As we noted earlier, children, of 5 to 9 years are fascinated by ritual. If they are not included, an important part of the grieving process may be missing for them. Exclusion from a family activity and the opportunity to share memories and meanings of the event could hinder their grief and cause resentment at a later date. However, some parents do not feel comfortable with including children in the funeral. They may have other ways of sharing and making meaning out of the experience with their children. Siblings describe their experience:

At the end, while I was crying, my little cousin came up to me and gave me a hug and said it was OK. She was only three. (Worden 1996, p. 22)

Anybody who wanted to could come. It is for children too, a way for little kids to understand that people have a life on earth but they die. (Teenage boy; Worden 1996, p. 22)

Everyone gave me support. It made me feel better that all the people were there. (Teenage girl; Worden 1996, p. 22)

There was a big funeral. All his school friends turned up ... I can still remember this feeling of detachment watching the coffin go off, with, on top, this expensive electric guitar he'd bought. ... I was more concerned with my parents and sister and I detached myself from my own emotions. I felt this responsibility to keep it all together. (Bereaved sister; Farrant 1998, p. 98)

In Donnelly's book (1982, p. 79) Stephanie Allen's experience was that: '*She felt she shouldn't be crying at her brother's funeral. There were more than a thousand people there, and Stephanie worked so hard to keep it all inside that she could never break*

through that wall again. ... At the funeral she felt that if she cried, she would be expos-
ing part of herself to all those people'.

BEHAVIOURAL REACTIONS OF CHILDREN TO THE DEATH OF A SIBLING

In Dent et al (1996) and Dent (2000), parents were asked what behavioural changes (if any) they had noticed in surviving children since the death of their child. Despite their own grief, the parents identified a range of changes (Table 4.1).

Behavioural changes noted by the parents included children being 'clingy', needing more attention than before, showing off and having sleep disturbances. It was noted that children in the second study, who had been bereaved 6 months, showed a higher percentage of behavioural changes than those who had been bereaved from 9 months to 2 years. It would appear that the likelihood of behavioural changes increases in the first 6 months after a death, especially in the form of aggression. Whether these behavioural difficulties produce long-term effects is unclear.

Immediate and short-term reactions can include problems at school caused by poor concentration and increased aggression (Pettle & Britten 1995). Sometimes the opposite happens and children will use school as an escape from the family and home (Kandt 1994). Children at all ages can show different forms of regressive behaviour (Dyregrov 1991). Any changes in behaviour can provide insights into children's emotional state and coping (Fleming & Balmer 1991).

Worden (1996) suggested that most disturbed behaviours are short lived and cease without any intervention. The focus should not be on the presence of a symptom but on its duration. He noted that there are several indicators that point to the need for further investigation:

- a child who has persistent difficulty in talking about their dead sibling
- aggressive behaviour that becomes worse and is destructive
- anxiety that persists, so that a child becomes clingy and/or exhibits school phobia.

Table 4.1
Behavioural changes in children since the death of a sibling

Characteristics	Study 1 (Dent et al 1996)	Study 2 (Dent 2000)
Study parameters		
No.	68	82
Age	10 months to 15 years	1 week to 12 years
Time since death	9 months to 2 years	6 months
Behavioural changes (%)		
Becoming withdrawn	39	43
Aggressive	25	65
Bed-wetting	18	25
Telling fibs	21	37
Being bullied	14	16
Unable to concentrate	21	38

It would seem natural to expect that when a sibling dies, and the whole family is in a state of confusion, surviving children will react in some way. This raises several questions. Can it be assumed that bereaved siblings will inevitably experience a time of disturbed behaviour? Do these symptoms arise as a result of the bereavement and/or changes in the functioning of the family or because their needs are not being met? Do behavioural changes occur in families where there is open communication, where information and choices are given to surviving children and where their feelings are acknowledged and understood? Are bereaved children who experience behavioural difficulties more, or less, likely to experience problems in later life? For those who exhibit no behavioural changes, are they more likely to have difficulties in later life? Such questions demonstrate that there is a need for further well-constructed research in this area.

CHILDREN'S FEELINGS ABOUT FAMILY AND OTHERS

Many of the children with whom Riches and Dawson (2000) worked expressed feelings of being left out, ignored and isolated within the family. Riches and Dawson (2000, p. 77) wrote, '*The key message we hear over and over is that bereaved siblings feel they are overlooked*'. Parents made similar comments; hence the title of their book *An intimate loneliness*.

> *I feel our family is not whole and never will be until we all die. We don't go out as much or go camping. We're usually locked in our rooms. I feel confused, scared and I always wonder what will happen to us or to me. I hope my family can become whole again.* (Priscilla aged 12; Silverman 2000, p. 158)

> *I hated our house, but they would come over and say 'Be with your mother. Try to help her'. They just never understood. I didn't have enough strength to help her. I needed all my energy to go to school.* (10-year-old boy; Sarnoff Schiff 2000, p. 89)

> *I felt like I had been pushed aside and I used to cry in my bedroom. I wanted to be talked to as a person, but instead I felt like a burden every time I tried to speak to my parents about Robbie. The thing I wanted most was my parents' time, so we could talk, but that rarely happened. Instead, our house seemed like it was always filled with people.* (Bereaved sibling; Sarnoff Schiff 1977, p. 86)

> *I was very worried about how my parents were feeling and felt that if I ever let all my sadness and grief show, it would make things worse for them. I never talked to them about my feelings.* (Bereaved sibling; Rosen 1986, p. 17)

However, when explanations are given, and a child is involved in rituals, there may be less likelihood of isolation.

> *I didn't remember having anyone close to me die. I was pretty good for a couple of days because I thought after a few days he was coming back to life. ... I looked everywhere for him. I didn't really understand. Now I am glad Mum and Dad explained everything about what was going on and they took me to the wake and the funeral.* (5-year-old Mark; Silverman 2000, p. 153)

MAKING MEANING OF THE DEATH

Like parents, children need to make meaning of the death. Much will depend on what the lost relationship has meant to them. The ages of the surviving children and how they characterise their connection to the dead child may vary. Younger children may see the death as a lack of playmate or competitor, while older children may feel they have lost a role model, a protector or a friend. Riches and Dawson (2000) suggested that opportunities for open and effective communication lie at the heart of children's successful adaptation to the death. The more family members talk about the death, the greater the chances of children being able to make sense of their experience. When the death is 'invisible', as in miscarriage, this may be more difficult for parents. Everyday activities may help a child to express feelings, fears and anxieties, so that insights are gained and some meaning made. The value of stories for adults making meaning has been indicated in the work of Nadeau (1998). Contributors to the book edited by Smith and Pennells (1985) emphasised the value of enabling children to express their feelings and this may include telling their stories. This can be verbal or graphic. Many younger children enjoy drawing and much can be learnt by listening to their explanation of their work and their perception of the death.

There are now many books written for children of varying ages. While books can be a useful tool, they are not a substitute for careful listening. They can be prompters for discussion, especially with younger children, to talk about their ideas and feelings surrounding their sibling's death. The main value of books is to provide a platform to initiate further discussion. Various techniques have been developed to help bereaved children. Many can be found in *Interventions with bereaved children* (Smith & Pennells 1995) and *Working with bereaved children* (Lindsey & Elsegood 1996).

CONSTRUCTING A RELATIONSHIP WITH THE DEAD SIBLING

Just as many parents find ways of remembering their dead child, some siblings need to find ways of maintaining ongoing attachments to the dead brother or sister. Hogan and DeSantis (1992) proposed that there are several ways of doing this. Surviving children dream, think about and talk to the deceased. Coles (1996) found that there were ongoing conversations in which the siblings shared feelings and expressed regret about things not done. As one sibling described (Silverman 2000, p. 165), '*I told him how I miss him, things about school and that I changed schools so I could be with my best friends*'.

Creating tokens of remembrance

Children may benefit from having their own tokens of remembrance of their dead sibling. A photograph, some special toy, a photograph album of pictures of the deceased child with the family, a scrapbook or a memory box may remind them that their sibling lived and is still part of their family. Some children may want to look at photographs over and over again (Silverman 2000).

There are a lot of memories that I can't share with anyone else. I'd love to sit and talk with him about old times. Sometimes I do talk with him. (Bereaved sibling aged 17 years; Silverman 2000, p. 155)

We planted a miniature rose in our school garden in memory of Natalie. (Ward 1996, p. 57)

Today I didn't cry. The pages of your scrapbook stayed dry. As I turned the pages, you came back to me and we played at the park and I laughed at the ducks. I pushed your pram down the sidewalk and we giggled at the birds. We had birthday cake and chased leaves together. As I turned the pages, you and I lived again … we were brother and sister. (11-year-old Alicia; Sims 1986, p. 38)

Having memories or tokens helps children to have a continuing bond with their deceased sibling (Klass 1996). This will mean finding a way to construct a changed relationship with them. Although the dead child is physically absent, surviving children need to be able to contemplate their lives with warmth and affection rather than with a sense of overwhelming distress (Rubin 1984). However, not all children may want tokens of remembrance. Anger, resentment and jealousy towards their dead sibling may prevent them from wanting reminders.

ARE THERE DIFFERENCES BETWEEN BEREAVED BOYS AND GIRLS?

The literature on gender differences in grieving children is very limited, although Dyregrov (1991) found that many bereaved parents spontaneously mentioned differences in this area. As we discussed in Chapter 2, such differences may reflect cultural expectations of gender-appropriate behaviour. Alternatively, as one bereaved sister described, family experiences may shape behaviours regardless of gender (Silverman 2000, p. 158). '*I'm like my father. I don't cry. I am very bothered when I see my mother cry. I want to run away from the pain … Sometimes I go visit a friend.*'

Worden (1996) suggested that more boys than girls refrain from talking about the death and have more difficulty in showing their feelings. Dyregrov (1991) cited his 1988 study of boys' and girls' reactions to the murder of a schoolteacher. He noted that girls were more likely than boys to acknowledge grief and crisis reactions, cry, experience difficulty concentrating and become jumpy or anxious. By comparison, boys tried to control their thoughts and feelings. Girls could write extensively about their first reactions while the boys gave short answers and showed little ability to translate their feelings into words. He also found that support varied; the majority of girls had a good friend in whom to confide, but only 40% of the boys reported the same. In addition, more girls had talked about the event at home than boys. Worden (1996) also reported differences between girls and boys. He proposed that girls are more affected by the death of a sibling than boys. In particular, he found that adolescent girls whose sibling had died showed higher levels of anxiety, depression and attention problems than adolescent girls who had lost a parent. As we described in Chapter 2, such findings suggest that individuals respond to, and make meaning of, death in different ways.

THE IMPACT OF SIBLING BEREAVEMENT

Studies indicate that sibling grief can be profound and long lasting in many cases, exerting a significant influence on adult mental health (Hindmarch 1995, Segal et al 1995). Black (1996) suggested that bereaved siblings have a higher risk of psychiatric disorders in later childhood and adult life, with a greater tendency to depression when the death was traumatic. However, Harrington and Harrison (1999) argued that childhood bereavement is not a major risk factor for mental and behavioural disorder in either childhood or adult life. One of the few longitudinal studies of adolescents was conducted between 7 and 9 years after the death of a sibling from cancer (Martinson & Campos 1991); it concluded that around one in six children still believed their sibling's death continued to have a major and negative impact on their lives. They still avoided talking about it for fear of upsetting their parents.

However, Riches and Dawson (2000) and Heiney (1991) noted that negative consequences are not inevitable. It is how the family as a whole copes with the death that determines the quality of the surviving children's adjustment. Giving information, explanations, involving them in rituals and providing opportunities to share feelings may increase likelihood of a bereaved child making sense of the death. As Pettle and Britten (1995) described, early recognition of children's grief and opportunities to explore and express feelings can prevent long-term difficulties. When there is an atmosphere of loving, respect and care, then children are more likely to express their fears, feelings and anxieties more readily (Hogan & DeSantis 1992). Children will also take cues from their parents as to how to grieve. The family context can shape their experience positively or negatively. The work of several researchers indicates that themes within the lives of some bereaved siblings include lack of parental attention and being placed in the role of passive observers (Rubin 1996, Riches & Dawson 2000, Rosenblatt 2000).

Segal et al (1995) posit that the nearer the deceased child was in age to the surviving children, the greater will be their sense of identification. In the case of an older child's death, or of children who died before the sibling was born, identity difficulties may arise (Powell 1995). Simon, now in his early forties, remembered that as a child he felt dogged by the feeling that he was inferior to the brother who had died at birth several years before he was born (Farrant 1998, pp. 16–17).

I had this deep-centred sense of inferiority and I felt the need to prove to my parents that I could be as good as this other child might have been. No one in the family ever talked openly about him. In fact, I've never been told officially of his existence. I can see with hindsight that there was no way that my mother should possibly have imagined that the fact that she had had a stillborn child would affect me ... what affected me was the image I constructed, not the fact of his death. ... I just picked up clues, if you like. And my creation was this paragon brother. I can see that secrets are often kept for the best reasons and it's done with good intent. But from my experience, sometimes it backfires.

Hogan and Desantis (1994) concluded that many siblings do progress from a highly vulnerable position during bereavement to have a greater self-awareness and maturity. There is some evidence to show that, for some children, bereavement may have long-lasting sequelae for psychological and social well-being (McCown & Pratt 1985, Rubin 1996). For other children, the experience may bring emotional growth and appreciation of the value of life (Hogan & DeSantis 1994). As one sibling described (Rosen 1986, p. 67):

I now live each day as if it may be someone's last. I won't part with anyone in anger; I want to leave them knowing that I care. I think I have become a more caring person because of my experience. I am a better listener, and more considerate.

So, what helps bereaved siblings grieve? Riches and Dawson (2000) proposed that the primary role of health professionals after the death of a child is in helping parents to manage their own grief so that they feel nurtured and supported. If this can be achieved then there is more likelihood that they, in turn, will be able to support and nurture their surviving children. This is a reminder of the importance of the social and cultural contexts within which children live.

SOCIAL AND CULTURAL CONTEXTS

Shapiro (1996) described grief as a family developmental crisis, interwoven with the family's history and its current development, where the family's grief redirects their future life together. The capacity of surviving children to adapt successfully to sibling bereavement appears to be closely linked to the quality of their intimate relationships, both within the family and with outside support networks (Birenbaum et al 1989). Several researchers have argued that it may not be the death itself which affects a child longer term, but the changes and readjustments to the family system (Bradach & Jordan 1995, Black 1996, Rubin 1996).

The community that surrounds siblings includes family, friends and others. Some of these people may be unable to communicate with surviving siblings about the death of their brother or sister. This may occur for several reasons. People may need to construct a defence against their own death anxiety; avoiding the bereaved may be more comfortable. They may also believe that surviving siblings should be spared the pain of confrontation with death. Some individuals may respond out of a universally felt need to protect the social order from the potential chaos that loss creates (Rosen 1986). Others may be fearful of saying the wrong thing, of not knowing what to say, of upsetting the child; in which case it is better to say nothing. The fear of speaking the name of the deceased child may not just be confined to the bereaved family but also to the wider community.

Children of school age will spend a large part of each weekday with teachers and peers. Peers can share with and support each other. However, this is not always the case since bullying or being bullied can occur (Dent et al 1996, Dent 2000). Children may be helpful to each other in an informal way but as this may be their first encounter with death, they may look to their teachers for guidance and direction (Silverman 2000). Given the role of schools in children's lives, schools need protocols in place to respond to all deaths. Every teacher should be prepared to meet the needs of bereaved children (O'Toole 1991, Stevenson & Stevenson 1997).

PROVISION OF SERVICES TO BEREAVED CHILDREN

Over recent years there has been a continuing growth of services available to bereaved children. A wide range of activities are run by committed and trained personnel, offering varied activities to assist both children bereaved of a parent and a sibling, as well as their parent(s). Some services run groups for different ages or have individual sessions with the children. There are now well over 100 services in various parts of the UK. Many of them belong to the Child Bereavement Network (CBN), an umbrella organisation providing a resource to those working in the field. The CBN has established regular regional meetings for service providers to meet, learn, network and support each other. It provides a directory of all known services throughout the UK and supports providers with information on relevant issues, videos, yearly conferences and a newsletter. One of these services, Winston's Wish, conducted an evaluation of two camps held in Gloucestershire during May 1994 for bereaved children and their parent(s) (Stokes & Crossley 1995). Parents and children who had attended were visited at home and a semi-structured interview completed. Six main points were noted which indicated the perceived value of such support:

- children benefitted from the programme
- children's behaviour changed as a result of the camp in a positive way
- children were more open and settled
- children's understanding of death increased
- communication levels within the family improved
- children were helped to cope with their relative's death.

Stokes and Crossley (1995, p. 190) included the following comments from the children attending the camps:

> I learnt how to cope with it, I don't just remember the sad times … I remember the fun times. I used to cry every night, now I don't. I felt it was my fault, now I understand.

> I learnt about what happened to others, you knew it wasn't just you.

> I learnt it's alright to talk about it and it's not always a bad thing to cry.

However, the effects of such support on the experiences of bereaved siblings, as opposed to children bereaved of a parent, are unclear. Key performance indicators held by Winston's Wish note that:

- only 25% of children attending the camps had been bereaved siblings
- 10% of calls to the enquiry line have been about sibling loss
- the helpline received around 15% of all calls relevant to sibling bereavement (D Stubbs, personal communication, 2003).

As there are now many services for bereaved children, it may be that other resources are assisting bereaved siblings. Or perhaps parents and/or bereaved siblings are not accessing any resources? If so, is it because they are 'forgotten' and not being encouraged by family and friends to use available resources? Or do many siblings feel well supported by family and friends and do not feel a need for such resources? Such an explanation would seem to contrast with Riches and Dawson's (2000) work, which noted siblings' sense of *an intimate loneliness* within the family setting. It remains possible that family members and others overlook the grief of some bereaved siblings. However, until further information is available, firm conclusions cannot be drawn.

SUMMARY

At the beginning of the chapter, we questioned whether bereaved siblings were 'forgotten grievers'. From the comments made, it is clear that the response of children to a sibling death is influenced by their age and cognitive abilities as well as by their response to their parents' grief and the level of support that they receive from friends, school and the community.

SUMMARY POINTS

- The sibling role is an important one, so the death of a sibling is a major event in children's lives.
- Children's understanding of death will depend on their cognitive abilities, past death experiences and social and cultural influences.
- Surviving children appear to grieve in a similar way to adults but at younger ages may not be able to understand or express their feelings.
- Bereaved children may need opportunities to talk of the death and to be involved in family rituals if they choose to do so.
- The manner in which their parents cope with the death will influence the grieving of bereaved siblings.

REFERENCES

Altschul S 1988 Childhood bereavement and its aftermath (Emotions and Behaviour Monograph No. 8). International Universities Press, Madison CT

Bank S, Kahn MD 1982 The sibling bond. Basic Books, New York

Barnard P, Kane M 1995 Voices from the crowd: stories from the Hillsborough football stadium disaster. In: Smith C, Pennells M, (eds) Interventions with bereaved children. Jessica Kingsley, London, p 254–266

Birenbaum LK, Robinson MA, Phillips DS et al 1989 The response of children to the dying and death of a sibling. OMEGA, Journal of Death and Dying 20: 213–228

Black D 1996 Childhood bereavement. British Medical Journal 312: 1496

Bluebond-Langner M 1996. In the shadow of illness: parents and siblings of the chronically ill child. Princeton University Press, Princeton, NJ

Bradach KM, Jordan JR 1995 Long term effects of a family history of traumatic death on adolescent individuation. Death Studies 19: 315–336

Brent S, Speece M, Lin C et al 1996 The development of the concept of death among Chinese and US children 3–17 years of age: from binary to fuzzy concepts? OMEGA, Journal of Death and Dying 33: 67–83

Coles JE 1996 Enduring bonds: sibling loss in early childhood. School of Professional Psychology, University of Massachusetts, Boston, MA

Corr C 1984 Helping with death education. In: Wass H, Corr C (eds) Helping children cope with death: guidelines and resources. Hemisphere, New York, p 49–73

Davies B 1987 Family response to the death of a child: the meaning of memories. Journal of Palliative Care 3: 9–15

Davies B 1988a Shared life space and sibling bereavement responses. Cancer Nursing 11: 339–347

Davies B 1988b The family environment in bereaved families and its relationship to surviving sibling behaviour. Children's Health Care 17: 22–32

Davies B 1991 Long-term outcomes of adolescent sibling behaviour. Journal of Adolescent Research 6: 83–96

Dent A 2000 Support for families whose child dies suddenly from accident or illness. PhD thesis, School of Policy Studies, University of Bristol, UK

Dent A, Condon L, Fleming P et al 1996 A study of bereavement care after sudden and unexpected death. Archives of Disease in Childhood 74: 522–526

Donnelly KF 1982 Recovering from the loss of a child. Macmillan, New York

Dunn J, Plomin R 1990 Separate lives: why siblings are different. Basic Books, New York

Dyregrov A 1991 Grief in children: a handbook for adults. Jessica Kingsley, London

Farrant A 1998 Sibling bereavement: helping children cope with loss. Cassell, Cambridge, UK

Fleming S, Balmer L 1991 Group intervention with bereaved children. In: Papadatou D, Papadatos C (eds) Children and death. Springer, New York, p 105–124

Hallam B, Vine P 1996 Expected and unexpected loss. In: Lindsey B, Elsegood J (eds) Working with children in grief and loss. Ballière Tindall, London p 56–72

Harrington R, Harrison L 1999 Unproven assumptions about the impact of bereavement on children. Journal of the Royal Society of Medicine 92; 230–232

Heiney SP 1991 Sibling grief: a case report. Archives of Psychiatric Nursing 5: 121–127

Herbert M, Harper-Dorton KV 2002 Working with children, adolescents and their families. Blackwell, Oxford

Hindmarch C 1995 Secondary losses for siblings. Child: Care Health and Development 21: 425–431

Hitcham M 1995 Direct work techniques with the siblings of children dying from cancer. In: Smith S, Pennells M (eds) Interventions with bereaved children. Jessica Kingsley, London, p 24–44

Hogan N, DeSantis L 1992 Adolescent sibling bereavement: an ongoing attachment. Qualitative Health Research 2: 159–177

Hogan N, DeSantis L 1994 Things that help and hinder adolescent sibling bereavement. Western Journal of Nursing Research 16: 132–153

Kandt V 1994 Adolescent bereavement: turning a fragile time into acceptance and peace. School Counsellor 41: 203–211

Kenyon B 2001 Current research in children's conceptions of death: a critical review. OMEGA, Journal of Death and Dying 43: 63–91

Klass D 1996 The deceased child in the psychic and social worlds of bereaved parents during the resolution of grief. In: Klass D, Silverman P, Nickman S (eds) Continuing bonds. New understandings of grief. Taylor & Francis, Washington, DC, p 199–215

Lauer MF, Mulhern RK, Bohne JB et al 1985 Children's perceptions of their sibling's death at home to hospital: the precursors of differential adjustment. Cancer Nursing 8: 21–27

Lewis M, Schonfield D 1994 Role of child and adolescent psychiatric consultation and liaison in assisting children and their families in dealing with death. Child and Adolescent Psychiatric Clinic of North America 3: 613–627

Lindsey B, Elsegood J (eds) 1996 Working with children in grief and loss. Ballière Tindall, London

Lonetto R 1980 Children's conceptions of death. Springer, New York

Martinson I, Campos RG 1991 Adolescent bereavement: long-term responses to a sibling's death from cancer. Journal of Adolescent Research 6: 54–69

McCown D 1987 Factors related to bereaved children's behavioural adjustment. In: Barnes C (ed) Recent advances in nursing. Churchill Livingstone, London, p 89–93

McCown D, Pratt C 1985 Impact of children's behaviour. Death Studies 9: 323–335

Nadeau J 1998 Families making sense of death. Sage, Thousand Oaks, CA

Nagy M 1948 The child's theories concerning death. Journal of Genetic Psychology 73: 3–27

O'Toole D 1991 Growing through grief: a K-12 curriculum to help young people through all kinds of losses. Compassion Books, Burnville, NC

Pettle SA, Britten CM 1995 Talking with children about death and dying. Child: Care Health and Development 21: 395–404

Powell M 1995 Sudden infant death syndrome: the subsequent child. British Journal of Social Work 25: 227–240

Rando T 1986 The unique issues and impact of the death of a child. In: Rando T (ed) Parental loss of a child. Research Press, Champaign IL, p 3–44

Rando T 1989 Parental adjustment to the loss of a child. In: Papadatou D, Papadatos C (eds) Children and death. Hemisphere Publishing, New York, p 233–253

Raphael B 1994 Loss in adult life: the death of a child. In: Raphael B (ed) The anatomy of bereavement. Routledge, London, p 229–282

Rathbone B 1996 Developmental perspectives. In: Lindsey B, Elsegood J (eds) Working with children in grief and loss. Ballière Tindall, London, p 16–31

Riches G, Dawson P 2000 An intimate loneliness: supporting bereaved parents and siblings. Open University Press, Buckingham, UK

Robinson L, Mahon M 1997 Sibling bereavement: a concept analysis. Death Studies 21: 477–499

Rosen H 1986 Unspoken grief: coping with childhood sibling loss. Lexington Books, Toronto

Rosenblatt P 2000 Parents' grief: narratives of loss and relationship. Brunner/Mazel, Philadelphia, PA

Rubin S 1984 Mourning distinct from melancholia: the resolution of bereavement. British Journal of Medical Psychology 57: 339–345

Rubin S 1996 The wounded family: bereaved parents and the impact of adult child loss. In: Klass D, Silverman P, Nickman S (eds) Continuing bonds. New understandings of grief. Taylor & Francis, Washington, DC, p 217–234

Sarnoff Schiff H 1977 The bereaved parent. Souvenir Press, London

Segal N, Wilson SM, Bouchard TJ, Gitlin DG 1995 Comparative grief experiences of bereaved twins and other bereaved relatives. Personality and Individual Differences 18: 511–524

Shapiro E 1996 Family bereavement and cultural diversity: a social developmental perspective. Family Process 35: 313–332

Silverman P 2000 Never too young to know. Oxford University Press, New York

Sims A 1986 Am I still a sister? Big A, Albuquerque, NM

Smith SC, Pennells M (eds) 1995 Interventions with bereaved children. Jessica Kingsley, London

Speece MW 1984 Children's understanding of death: a review of three components of a death concept. Child Development 55: 1671–1986

Stevenson RG, Stevenson EP 1997 Teaching students about death. Charles Press, Philadelphia, PA

Stewart A 2000 When an infant grandchild dies: family matters. PhD thesis, School of Nursing, University of Wellington, Wellington NZ

Stokes J, Crossley D 1995 Camp Winston: a residential intervention for bereaved children. In: Smith S, Pennells M (eds) Interventions with bereaved children. Jessica Kingsley, London, p 172–193

Walter T 1996 A new model of grief: bereavement and biography. Mortality 1: 7–27

Ward B 1996 Good grief: exploring feelings, loss, and death with over elevens and adults – a holistic approach Jessica Kingsley, London

Wass H 1984 Concepts of death: a developmental perspective. In: Wass H. Corr C (eds) Childhood and death. Hemisphere, Washington, DC, p 3–24

Worden JW 1996 Children and grief. Guildford Press, New York

USEFUL SOURCES FOR NURSES AND MIDWIVES

Hindmarch C 2000 On the death of a child, 2nd edn. Radcliffe Medical Press, Oxford

Lindsey B, Elsegood J (eds) 1996 Working with children in grief and loss. Ballière Tindall, London

Riches G, Dawson P 2000 An intimate loneliness: supporting bereaved parents and siblings. Open University Press, Buckingham

Silverman P 2000 Never too young to know. Oxford University Press, Oxford

Smith C, Pennells M (eds) 1995 Interventions with bereaved children. Jessica Kingsley, Publishers, London

Family bereavement: the experience of grandparents

> *I truly believe there can be nothing more sorrowful in our lives. My agony is for my son and his wife; the terrible emptiness for them. I would do anything to make it easier for them. I am never quite sure which makes me more desolate, the child's death or her parents' sorrow.*
>
> Grandmother writing about the death of her 9-year-old granddaughter from cancer; Ponzetti and Johnson 1991, p. 164

> *In my grief, I feel the loss of a little boy coming here to see me. The loss that he is not here to share the birthdays and the Christmases and the Mother's Days.*
>
> Catherine talking about the death of her grandson Samuel

INTRODUCTION

The words of these grandmothers are about the enormity of experiencing a grandchild die during childhood. They describe the meaning that this has for their relationships, roles and shared experiences within the family. In 'Setting the scene', we described the death of a child creating a *'death ripple'* that flows into the family and community (Jordan et al 1993, p. 425). The focus of other people's attention is generally on the parents, who are at the centre of the ripple. The grief of other people touched by the extending ripples may not be recognised. Hence, grandparents have been called *'forgotten grievers'* in the titles of articles (Gyulay 1975, Ponzetti & Johnson 1991). So, what are grandparents' experiences of grief? Are grandparents forgotten? And if so, by whom? This chapter explores these questions.

THE CONTEXT OF THIS CHAPTER

The content in this chapter includes stories of grandparents and parents, research and our experience from clinical practice. As we discussed in Chapter 2, grief is diverse. It has different meanings for individual grandparents. This is illustrated by Jenny's story (Box 5.1) and the comments from other grandparents about the experience of having a grandchild die suddenly. The discussion in this chapter

Box 5.1 Jenny's story

Who am I?

I am a grandmother whose first long-awaited grandson, Jordan, was stillborn just 3 weeks before the expected 'due' date, Of course our family and friends have been really supportive but when I'm asked, 'How are you?' or 'How are you feeling?' I don't know how to answer.

How did I feel?

When I arrived at the hospital and was taken into a darkened room to be with Susie and Charlie and told their baby was dead, I knew how I felt then. Pain, such pain and an over-powering love for my daughter and son-in-law, and the need to try and 'make everything alright again for them'. Initially, I felt physically sick and faint – knowing my darling grandson was about to be born, knowing the total silence that follows will be so painful. Instead of a crying, breathing bundle of joy, they would be seeing a still and silent baby – so very still, I needed to be with them. We got to the ward at 3:25 a.m. to find Susie sitting up in bed and trying to smile, to make us all feel better. ... When we were able to hold our grandson, it was wonderful to look on his beautiful face and touch his tiny fingers but I felt I wanted to breathe life into him. I knew it had no way of making any difference but he only looked asleep. The urge to sing a lullaby to my first born little grandson, Jordan, as I'd done for his mother when she was newborn, was almost too much to bear.

Box 5.1
Continued

Jordan's funeral

The chapel at our local crematorium was filled by family and friends and many work colleagues. Charlie carried Jordan's tiny coffin and placed a musical soft toy (a present from Jordan's proposed god-parents) on top of the casket. I placed a single cream rose on his coffin. A tape of dolphin music was played. This was very special to Susie while she was expecting Jordan. The piece was 'Ave Maria'. It was so beautiful with the sounds of the dolphins against the noise of the crashing waves. We left the chapel after singing 'All things bright and beautiful'. This was Charlie's choice – he wanted people leaving with the feeling of hope, not despair. ...

How did I feel?

We had all been focusing on Jordan's funeral wanting to do small, special things for him: choosing flowers, music, the service format, knowing this would be our only chance of giving of ourselves to our very special little person. Close family and friends came back to our bungalow after the service, and, with the help of Charlie's Mum, I prepared a buffet lunch, which we ate in the garden. This was a continuation of our giving, by helping our children in any way possible. Once Jordan's ashes had been interred, instead of the comfort of knowing everything had been completed I felt nothing was left 'to see to'. That there was a dark, gaping hole before me.

How do I feel nearly 8 months on?

I feel a double pain. The despair of seeing my own child suffering so badly and also the hollow emptiness of a grandmother whose dreams of holding and nursing her daughter's baby going unfulfilled. I call myself Jordan's nanny but then a voice in my head says, 'You're not really a nanny yet'. But part of me says 'I am'. So, what am I? Where do we go from here? The 'bottom line' is I feel so many things, but mainly I feel confused and isolated in my grief, and still carrying so much pain.

How do I feel 2 years later?

It's well over 2 years since Jordan's death and of course we have travelled a long way emotionally. I still feel pain when I see my friends with their lovely grandchildren or Nannies pushing their grandchild about on the green or at our superstore. I have a lot of 'If only's' still to conquer. So I try to be positive and thank God for my children and their happy marriages, the love they share and their good health and prospering careers.

What about grief as a grandparent?

If asked about grief 10 years ago, I'd not experienced any so I would have felt it was like a great sadness and one that can be lived through relatively easily on a day-to-day basis. But I now know how different every loss is; how all encompassing, how dark and miserable each day can seem, how

Box 5.1
Continued

you can cease to function emotionally but also how physically ill you can become. When a child like Jordan dies, you feel impotent to find any answers to the many questions we asked and that our children asked. We feel cheated by something that can't be expressed. We did talk and share our feelings at the beginning because speaking about Jordan seemed to make him a reality and not a dream. But I didn't talk about my own feelings as a grandma. My feelings and needs seemed less important than Jordan's parents so I put myself second for a long while.

Memories and anniversaries
With a stillbirth there are no memories as you'd have with an older grandchild, so the photos and letters and cards are very important. Susie and Charlie have also been given a photo, hair and footprint from the maternity home and these are very special to them. I always think of Jordan when I see candles alight. A family friend wrote a small verse in her sympathy card that has stayed with me ever since: ' A little candle, never lit. Yet still shines in the dark.'

Also, Jordan was with us so briefly that his spirit seemed transient to me. On the first anniversary of losing him I took a blue balloon, with lots of streamers, down to the Garden of Rest. And told Jordan how much we loved and missed him and that Nanny and Granddad couldn't hug him so we were sending our love up to him – I kissed the balloon and let it float up and away.

cannot be assumed to apply to all grandparents. The majority of this chapter, including comments from named grandparents and parents, comes from the research in which Jenny participated and which was described on page xii (Stewart 2000). Excerpts from this work are presented in this chapter. Reference is also made to four other research studies that have contributed to knowledge about grandparent bereavement. DeFrain, Jakub and Mendoza (1991–2) received replies to a questionnaire mailed to 80 American grandparents, of whom 64 were grandmothers whose grandchild died of sudden infant death syndrome (SIDS). Ponzetti and Johnson (1991) undertook a similar descriptive study of 45 bereaved American grandparents, of whom 34 were grandmothers. The majority of grandchildren died from illness or cancer, which meant that there was some forewarning of death. In a further study, Ponzetti (1992) compared the reactions of 36 American parents and 28 grandparents. They were family members of 21 children aged 1 month to 30 years who died for various reasons, not all of which were unexpected. More recently, Fry (1997) undertook a study with two phases. In the first, 152 American grandparents completed a questionnaire about having a grandchild die for any reason aged 6–32 years. In the second, 17 grandparents, of whom 12 were grandmothers, were interviewed during the 6 months after their grandchild's death.

THE GRIEF OF GRANDPARENTS

What can we learn from Jenny's story and other perspectives of grandparent bereavement? Jenny's story highlighted the ways in which her grandson's death challenged and changed her life forever. Aspects of this experience include the untimeliness of death, the relationship that grandparents hold with the parents and the ways in which grandparents cope and find ways to live with the death. These issues arise in the experiences of some other grandparents and also formed part of the discussion in Chapter 2.

THE DEATH OF A GRANDCHILD IS UNTIMELY AND DEVASTATING

Shock and disbelief are common reactions to the news of a sudden death, which turns the family world upside down. Catherine described her memory of the day after Samuel's death. '*I can remember the next day the milkman was coming and the paper was delivered and I thought, "Why were all these things still happening?" Because the world had stopped for us.*' Death of a grandchild is unexpected even when grandparents are aware that children do die suddenly. Ailsa explained '*it's something you think will happen to somebody else and not that you or your family will be affected*'. Most importantly, as the family lifecycle in Chapter 1 indicates, such a death is outside the expected course of events where grandparents die before their grandchildren. This can create a sense of '*grave untimeliness*' (Fry 1997, p. 128). For some grandparents, this can lead to feelings of anger or guilt. Anger may be framed around the question '**Why** did my grandchild die with no opportunity to fulfil their potential?' and be directed towards the world, particular people or even God (DeFrain et al 1991–2). Other grandparents grapple with the question '**Why** not me instead? I'm older, I would have taken their place'. Many grandparents in Fry's research identified such feelings of survival guilt, although this has not been the case in other research studies (Ponzetti & Johnson 1991, Ponzetti 1992, Stewart 2000). Other feelings of guilt may exist. For example, DeFrain et al (1991–2) found that 29% of 80 American grandparents of children with SIDS expressed feelings of personal guilt regarding responsibility for the baby's death, either because of particular actions or a belief that they could have prevented it.

One of the main findings of the study of DeFrain et al (1991–2, p. 165) was that a grandchild's death was a '*devastating experience*' that affected all aspects of grandparents' lives. The effects can include a wide range of physical changes such as altered sleep patterns, loss of appetite, weight loss, diarrhoea, inability to remember things and fatigue (DeFrain et al 1991–2, Ponzetti 1992, Stewart 2000). Existing health conditions such as angina or arthritis may be exacerbated. Some grandparents attribute physical symptoms to the bereavement (Ponzetti & Johnson 1991). Others, as Jenny described, focus on the parents' grief and this may preclude recognition of the physical stresses of their own grief.

BEREAVED GRANDPARENTS AS PARENTS OF THE PARENTS

One of the unique elements of grandparents' grief is their role in relation to the grandchild. This is as parents of the parents of the grandchild. Benita, whose grandson died, described hearing the phrase '*being parents first*', at a conference. This captures the central focus of many grandparents' grief, described by Jenny as the pain that she felt for her daughter and son-in-law. Grandparents' concern and pain for the parents of the child are reported in all the research studies. Gyulay (1975, p. 1478) referred to this as '*triple-layered grief*'. Grief for the parent, for self and for the grandchild. Marie said, '*You have got all those extra ones to grieve for when you are a grandmother*'. Elisabeth wrote, 3 years after her grandson Martin died, about the overwhelming intensity of this multiple grief.

> *Grief took on a whole new meaning after Martin died, the double grief was almost unbearable – watching our own child and her husband. And feeling the loss of our grandson. It seemed so enormous and as a person who was usually in control of my public emotions I suddenly found I would weep in the most unexpected places and with the most unexpected people – this was difficult and hard to accept.*

As Rando (1986, p. 37) observed, grandparents '*not only lose their grandchild but they "lose" their child as well, as they cannot rescue their child from bereaved parent status*'. This situation can create feelings of helplessness (DeFrain et al 1991–2, Ponzetti & Johnson 1991, Fry 1997) which Ailsa, the grandmother of Conor, described:

> *I think, for me, one of the hardest parts was seeing my children so devastated and not being able to do anything for them. Because when your children are little you can fix all their aches, or all their problems. And as they get older their problems get bigger and you can do less about them. And there is nothing you can do to make it better for them and this is worse than anything else.*

While unable to 'fix' the situation, many grandparents respond to the death of a grandchild by going to be with the parents, offering help and showing that they care.

HELPING OUT BUT NOT TAKING OVER

The role of parent of the bereaved parents can be a complex and difficult one (Stewart 2000). Many grandparents, like Jenny and Ailsa, describe wanting to be with, help and support the bereaved parents. However, such offers of help are generally mindful that the grandparent's child is an adult in their own right. This means helping out but not taking over from the parents of the dead child. Keith explained that this needs sensitivity. '*You are trying to help them and you really have to be very careful. They have to be left to do what they want to do. But you can see things that you could probably help with – but check it with them*.'

Help can include practical advice on organising a funeral, cooking meals and caring for other children. It may extend to offering financial assistance towards the costs of the funeral or a headstone. For many grandparents 'being with' the parents is a central part of helping out. It involves sharing time together, offering comfort and companionship by sometimes talking and sometimes listening. Such activities enable surviving family members to restructure relationships with each other in the changed family world (Fry 1997).

While many grandparents spend time with the bereaved parents, other grandparents are unable to do so for a range of reasons. These include physical and mental illness, geographical distances separating the families and estrangement between family members. In many instances, practical advice and emotional support are still offered through regular telephone calls or emails. When it is not, the grief of grandparents may have a different meaning to that of grandparents who keep in contact with the bereaved parents and other siblings.

WHAT HELPS GRANDPARENTS COPE AND LIVE WITH THE DEATH OF A GRANDCHILD?

Bereaved grandparents, like people experiencing other losses, seek to cope with the stresses caused by a sudden, unexpected death. They then find a way to live with the meaning of the death and the effect it has on the family. In the second study by Fry (1997, p. 132), the 17 grandparents said '*their first priority was to support their adult children and their families, and to re-engage in family activities that were part of their lives prior to the grandchild's death*'. Stewart (2000) found a similar pattern. Grandparents constructed the death of a grandchild as a challenge. This challenge needed a short-term response of helping and caring for the parents. In the long-term, grandparents managed the challenge of making sense of the loss and reorganising family relationships. This included talking, keeping busy and using previous experiences and information to understand the experience. Similarly, Fry (1997, p. 135) found '*grandmothers and grandfathers struggle individually to make personal choices regarding coping measures they felt were best for them*'.

INFORMATION CAN HELP

For many grandparents, having knowledge about what is happening and what choices are available, can help them to cope with the situation. Information is often combined with personal experiences of loss in order to gain insights and identify ways to help the parents cope. Beth commented after reading 'Grandparents and holidays' in Gerner's book (1990):

It touched a chord as Christmas came not long after Daniel's death. We floundered through. This book would have been helpful at the time. It has helped me now with Daniel receiving a gift at Christmas time, as does everyone else. It is a decoration for the tree to remember him by. It is much appreciated by his parents and will continue.

While personal experience of previous loss can assist grandparents to cope, if there are multiple losses in a short period of time it can result in '*bereavement overload*' (Moss & Moss 1997, p. 4). Such overload has the potential to happen to any family member. However, grandparents, as older people, may be more likely to experience multiple bereavements with the deaths of friends and spouses. In addition, the death of a grandchild may lead some grandparents to revisit their personal experience of having a baby or child die. They may decide to mark the place of their own dead child using opportunities that may not have been available at the time that their own child died. For example, writing their name in a book of remembrance or attending a candlelight service. For a few grandparents, previous experiences of death or loss may mean that they have difficulty coping with their grief after a grandchild's death. This may limit the support that they feel able to offer the bereaved parents and may even result in the parents trying to support the grandparent (Stewart 2000).

COPING AS CARING

Many grandparents find that caring is one way of coping (Stewart 2000). This includes offering practical and emotional help to the parents at the time of death and subsequently (Fry 1997). Catherine talked about the benefits of helping.

> *At the time Samuel died I felt, not necessarily useful, but that I was able to be of some help and I think that helped that feeling of helplessness. It was a little highlight when I was able to do something for my daughter and son-in-law, like a phone call.*

Funerals offer an opportunity for grandparents to help parents and thus show their care for the parents and their child. Many grandparents, like Jenny, assist parents with a range of decisions involved in organising a funeral such as location, choice of music, words, activities and symbols. The funeral provides a ritual, which is a farewell to the grandchild. It also provides a shared activity for family members, with opportunities to talk, cry and share memories. This can begin the process of reconstructing the family world. In the long term, some grandparents find that helping people in the local community can offer a way of making meaning from the death (DeFrain et al 1991–2, Fry 1997, Stewart 2000).

TALKING AND KEEPING BUSY

Many grandparents appreciate opportunities to talk about their experience. Talking can help to share memories, make sense of the experience and reconstruct a view of the changed family world. Fry (1997, p. 131) found that a number of grandparents '*spoke of their reminiscing and remembering the past and reconciling it with the present as a way of recovering from grief*'. While broad gender differences may exist, with grandmothers more likely to talk than grandfathers (DeFrain et al 1991–2), individual differences are equally apparent (Stewart 2000). Not all grandparents want to talk; some find other ways of coping with their grief as Elisabeth confided. '*Writing has helped me greatly to come to terms with Martin's death. I enjoy writing his name.*' Writing his name provided a story that became a memorial to him and which has become available publicly in a booklet for bereaved families produced by the Stillbirth and Neonatal Death Society (SANDS), Aberdeen.

Regardless of whether grandparents talk about their experience, many agree that they cope by keeping busy, either caring for the bereaved parents or involved in work or household activities. This description appears to reflect the alternation between loss- and restoration-orientated coping that Stroebe and Schut (2001) described in the dual process model (p. 29). As Marie described, using different coping strategies can make the pain manageable. '*There are sometimes when it is just really too hard. I feel so sad for Rosemary and her family. And then I give myself a shake, get up and go and do something to take my mind off the pain.*'

MAKING SENSE OF THE EXPERIENCE

As parents described in Chapter 3, grandparents, too, face having to adjust to the death. One perspective is that this requires finding ways to make sense of the death in order to relearn, or reconstruct, an assumptive world. Death of a grandchild brings the primary loss of their presence and other losses according to the meaning that being a grandparent holds for each individual.

The meaning of a grandchild's death

A grandparent's relationship and role within the family influences the meaning that the death holds. Numerous factors such as age, employment, geographic proximity, relationship with the parents and ethnic group can shape grandparents' activities with their family (Barranti 1985, Hurme 1991, Smith 1991). Many grandparents enjoy the role, which brings pleasures without the responsibilities of being a parent. Others, for various reasons, take on the role of surrogate parents (Fitzgerald 2001). Therefore, making sense of the experience is entangled with self-identity. Jenny described that the death of Jordan, her first-born grandchild, presented a question – was she **really** a grandmother? Conversely, when grandparents have more than one grandchild, then the gender of the dead grandchild may have a particular meaning. Alex and Benita had three sons, one of who was married with two daughters. Then a son, Matthew, was born. When Matthew died they felt the poignancy of the loss of an only grandson. The age of a grandchild can also bring a particular meaning to a grandparent's bereavement. When a baby is stillborn, or dies soon after birth, there are few memories or tokens of remembrance from their life or death. Conversely, as grandchildren grow up and develop their individual interests, these provide opportunities to develop special relationships with grandparents. Then the death can mean the loss of shared times together.

Ways of making sense

As we discussed in 'Setting the scene' and Section 1, people find their own ways to make sense of the experience using personal resources such as beliefs and values combined with social resources. Some grandparents have spiritual beliefs (Fry 1997) or a religious faith that offers a means to make sense of the experience (Ponzetti & Johnson 1991, Stewart 2000). However, in some instances, such beliefs do not help or are weakened by the death (DeFrain et al 1991–2, Ponzetti & Johnson 1991). Other grandparents hold a pragmatic philosophy of life. Ailsa described her view as '*what can't be cured must be endured*'. Similarly, previous experiences of death can offer both coping strategies and a way of making sense of the death. For the current generation of older people, this may include a sense of inevitability or a reserve about talking about death, having experienced the Second World War (Field 2000).

The terms 'getting over', 'accepting' or 'recovering' from a grandchild's death were not part of the experience of many grandparents (Stewart 2000). A number held the view that the world had changed and the bereavement was lifelong. Alex described his thoughts 4 years after Matthew's death. '*I don't think you ever completely get over it, but a major resolution has taken place. But there will always be occasions when it seems you go back into a space of coping with it, like anniversaries and that sort of thing.*' Interwoven with making sense of the death are the ways in which grandparents create relationships with their dead grandchild.

MARKING PLACE AND REMEMBERING THE GRANDCHILD

Parents undertake various activities to remember and maintain a relationship with their dead child (McClowry et al 1987, Riches & Dawson 1998). Grandparents too, construct a relationship with the dead grandchild. This includes revisiting memories as private thoughts and conversations with other family members, Sharing memories is also a way of helping existing and subsequent grandchildren to place themselves within the whole family. Ailsa, Conor's grandmother, described her role in this activity:

> We often talk about him. Not everyday conversation every day of the week, but we all do talk about Conor. In fact I was at Laurie and Suzanne's for tea last night and we were talking with Joanne [Conor's older sister] about it. The children were saying how they spelt his name and I said 'What was Conor's other name?' just in conversation. I think it is important for children, too, to bring that up now and again. Not just to push it away to the back.

Seeing tokens of remembrance often triggers memories. Like siblings, many grandparents appreciate having their own tokens of remembrance such as photographs, lock of hair, handprints, clothes, letters and toys. However, when a child dies around the time of birth there are limited opportunities to create such tokens of remembrance and these are generally 'owned' by the parents. This means that symbols, which offer a link to the grandchild, may be of particular importance to grandparents. For Jenny, candles symbolised Jordan, whereas Marie treasured an umbrella.

> Really, the only things I have to remember Ruby by are photos of her in her coffin, and strangely an umbrella. During the grave-side ceremony the rain was pouring down and I held this umbrella over the girls and me. This umbrella I will never use again but I have put it in a place I pass by most days and I touch it and remember.

Photographs of the child alive and/or dead can physically mark the place of the grandchild in the grandparents' home and life. Alex talked about photographs of his grandson Matthew. *'We keep them right in the middle of the family photographs which are on the wall as you go down the stairs, because we always want to feel that he is anchored very firmly [in the family]'.* Photographs are more than a tangible reminder of a missing family member, they are also a means of a continuing relationship, as Margaret explained. *'I would not want to be without the photograph on the wall, in the lounge and the bedroom. It is an image of Matthew that I can say, "Hello" to.'*

As Catherine indicated at the beginning of the chapter, family members remember the absence of a grandchild at family times. This includes Christmas, Father's Day, Mother's Day and the child's birth and death dates. Many grandparents have their own sadness at such times and mark the place of their dead grandchild. For Jenny, the release of a balloon marked a day to remember Jordan. At such times, some grandparents are uncertain whether to contact the parents or say nothing to avoid bringing up painful memories. Others recognise that many parents value the role that grandparents take to remember such dates with a phone call or by joining in a special family meal.

Most of the activities that maintain a continuing bond with the grandchild are undertaken by grandparents privately, with their partners or within the family. Sometimes grandparents are faced with a public dilemma. A commonplace question in everyday conversation is 'How many grandchildren **do** you have?' Grandparents use various strategies to reply, which include acknowledging all their grandchildren and sometimes differentiating between the number of living and dead. Elisabeth clearly marked the place of both her grandchildren:

> *I always say 'Two, but we lost the first grandchild, Martin, who was born too early and did not survive'. I like to mention his name. Then I go on to talk about Eilidh [Martin's sister] and bore the pants off them!*

An answer like Elisabeth's can stop the conversation momentarily, since the enquirer may be uncertain how to reply. As a result, some grandparents do not mention their dead grandchild as part of a conscious decision to avoid other people's discomfort. However, the importance placed by parents on including the child may lead some grandparents to change their reply, as Elwyn described:

> *When some-one asks me 'How many grandchildren do you have?' I count Daniel now. It was actually something my daughter-in-law said that made me stop and think. I have just became a member of Probus [retired professional and business women's group] and I had to give my profile. I went quickly through my life and said I had seven grandchildren. I gave it to my daughter-in-law to read and she actually pulled it up that I had missed Daniel out. Underneath it was probably because I didn't really know how to treat something like that and probably felt, 'well, I've got seven.' And I understood how she felt and I felt bad because it was almost like when she was reading she'd be thinking 'Oh he meant nothing'.*

RESOURCES TO ASSIST GRANDPARENTS

As we described in previous chapters, people use social resources from both within and outside the family to help them cope with death.

Within the family

Within some families, there is acknowledgement of a shared loss and the need for mutual support from parents to grandparents and vice versa (Stewart 2000). In other families, grandparents seek to offer support to parents without expecting support in return. Elisabeth wrote, '*I could share some feelings with Lorna and Geoff, but often I felt I must be strong for them and hide my feelings as they were struggling.*'

The focus of attention, by health professionals and others, on the parents may mean that even the parents may not immediately appreciate the extent of grandparents' grief. Rose described her experience. '*Because grandparents get completely forgotten in a grieving process when a family loses a child and nobody realises. I mean it took me a while to realise the depth of feeling that Mum and Dad have.*'

Many grandparents talk about feelings and memories with other family members such as own partner and particularly the mother of the child (DeFrain et al 1991–2). It provides emotional support and an opportunity to start reconstructing the changed family world (Stewart 2000). As we noted in Chapter 1, death creates a change to the existing family structure. It can change roles and relationships. Ponzetti (1992) found that 56% of parents and 53% of grandparents reported changes in their feelings to each other. In some situations, relationships can remain fragile or estranged and the assumption that a death 'brings the family together' is not apparent in some families (Stewart 2000).

Outside the family

Outside the family, acknowledgement of grandparents' grief may, or may not, be offered. Terese was hurt when '*other people would not talk to me*' at her workplace after her granddaughter Bernadette died. This mirrors parents' experiences described in Chapter 3 and often reflects the discomfort of other people at being with someone who is bereaved. Some grandparents describe being asked, '*how are … [the parents]?*' with accompanying comments such as '*It is a good thing that you are there for them*'. The intent of such comments is well meaning but carries a message that the grandparents' role is to support the parents and that their grief is more important. It can disenfranchise grandparents by removing a recognised space for their own grief. Jenny wrote about such lack of recognition:

> [I want] to be acknowledged by 'society and the media' to be suffering a great loss. Not just accepted as the 'tower of strength' for everyone else as the 'bottomless pit of experience' to be drawn on at will. But to be in need of a hug or a friendly ear, or just someone to sit and walk with in companionable silence.

Similar to the experiences of parents described in Chapter 3, many grandparents want people to phone, send cards and '*take the time to show they cared*' over the months and years following the death (DeFrain et al 1991–2, p. 180). While mutual help groups offer a place to talk and receive support, the majority of grandparents do not choose to attend such groups for a range of reasons (DeFrain et al 1991–2, Fry 1997), possibly because they have a focus on bereaved parents (Stewart 2000). The few grandparents who were contacted by a nurse, midwife or GP greatly appreciated the acknowledgement of their bereavement (Stewart 2000). While grandparents access some support from others, they form a large part of the support resources available to many bereaved parents. What do grandparents think helps the parents?

HOW CAN GRANDPARENTS HELP PARENTS AND OTHER CHILDREN?

When asked this question, Elisabeth made the following points based on her experience after Jordan's death:

- *Take your cue from the parents. Try to be helpful and understanding to their wishes – do not take away their responsibilities in any way. Allow time to mourn and express grief in the family and with friends when possible.*
- *Try to pave the way for friends and not-so-close family to share in the grief and understand how the parents feel.*
- *If the parents want to keep the lost baby's memory fresh and present, then bring the baby's name into the conversation. Remember birthdays, Christmas and other important family times.*
- *If there is a grave, visit it when you can. This lets the parents see that you remember every day, not just the special occasions.*

Some grandparents in the study of DeFrain et al (1991–2, p. 179) emphasised supporting the individuality of grief in relation to other family members with comments such as, '*If the grieving person wants to talk, cry or scream, let them do it. Just be there to listen, not to judge their actions*' and, '*To talk about the death is the best possible thing to do. Don't ignore the situation*'. Similar points about listening to parents are presented in the books written for grandparents either by a bereaved grandparent (Gerner 1990) or by people who have worked with bereaved grandparents (Leininger & Ilse 1985). Kolf (1995, pp. 21–22) proposed that grandparents remember the acronym of being a PAL:

- *Presence is about physically being there with the parents.*
- *Assistance is practical help.*
- *Listening whenever needed to parents talking through their 'tapes of grief' where the same story or feelings are repeated again and again.*

What do parents think helps? Most parents appreciate the practical and sometimes financial support that grandparents offer. Many see the support of grandparents as invaluable. Frazer described the experience of taking Matthew, his son, home to die. '*It would have been more of a nightmare for us, I think, without Mum and Dad there. I don't think we would have gone home on our own with just Sarah and me coping* with and holding Matthew and not knowing "Is he going to die?" or "Is he not going to die?".' Marie was unable to offer physical help because of arthritis, but Rose felt that Marie's advice helped her to cope after Ruby's death:

> She keeps my feet on the ground. When I moan about the girls [Ruby's older sisters] she says to me, 'You've got to be a bit more understanding' because sometimes I forget how deeply they've been affected by it. I mean you have a tendency to. I do know how badly they were affected but you tend to forget about it sometimes, because children appear so resilient and not say anything.

In contrast Pip, whose daughter died, wanted grandparents to include Gracie in family conversations. 'Grandparents have a role in remembering to remember. It is the **acknowledgement** that is important to me.'

ARE GRANDPARENTS FORGOTTEN GRIEVERS?

The previous discussion highlights that some parents may not immediately appreciate the nature and intensity of grandparents' grief. Hence they may be 'forgotten' in the short term by other family members. Yet, most parents appreciate and value the grief of grandparents because it indicates that the child was important (Stewart 2000). Outside the family, some grandparents may lack support and recognition from friends and colleagues, who focus on the role of grandparents as supporters to the parents. In addition, current societal values tend to marginalise older people and value youth (Moss & Moss 1997). This can mean that individuals, communities and health services forget grandparents' grief. Equally, some grandparents do not take the opportunity to claim their role as grievers. When asked how many grandchildren they have, a number choose not to indicate the death of their grandchild. This may avoid discomfort on the part of the enquirer but may not assist to make the place of grandparents' grief visible.

What about health professionals? Do they forget grandparents? Gyulay, a nurse working with American children who were terminally ill, wrote an article in 1975 entitled *The forgotten grievers*. She felt that four groups were overlooked by society and health professionals: fathers, siblings, grandparents and others such as peers and teachers. Sixteen years later Ponzetti and Johnson (1991) published a research study about grandparents with the same title. So 11 years still later, are grandparents still forgotten? Certainly in the years following 1975 the majority of writing and research in the fields of psychology, psychotherapy, counselling and health professionals' practice has focused on parents and siblings (see earlier chapters). There has been limited research with bereaved grandparents (e.g. DeFrain et al 1991–2, Ponzetti & Johnson 1991, Ponzetti 1992, Fry 1997, Stewart 2000) and few published clinical practice articles (e.g. Gerner 1988, Donnelly & Haimes 1993). The lack of comment, writing and research can mean that health professionals do not 'see' grandparents as people grieving who might want acknowledgement or support. Recently, Jane, a clinical nurse specialist in paediatrics, made this comment about her practice:

> *I do think grandparent bereavement is a very important, often overlooked issue. When a child dies, naturally everything is focused on the parents and siblings. However, grandparents are always so involved giving and just being there for the family. They are not just helping out with the meals; they are helping their children grieve. They are the ones left after a child dies providing support, listening and grieving themselves for the death of their grandchild and for the loss in their own children's lives. There would definitely be times where we could have, or should have, made contact with grandparents.*

As Jane described, many health professionals are aware of the support that grandparents offer the parents but can 'forget' the personal grief of grandparents when their point of contact, and focus of health service funding contracts, is the parents of the child. In some situations of practice, such as working in accident and emergency, the nature of the work may mean that it is 'rare' to meet grandparents. However, grandparent bereavement itself is not 'rare'.

SUMMARY

Health professionals need to be aware of the personal grief of grandparents in addition to acknowledging their roles as support for the parents. Increasingly, people are becoming great grandparents who will also be bereaved. Considering the extent of such grief and the role that grandparents take with grieving parents, we believe that nurses and midwives need to consider grandparents' grief as part of their practice after the sudden, unexpected death of a child.

SUMMARY POINTS

- Death of a child causes a ripple that leaves grandparents bereaved.
- Grandparents often live with a triple grief, which is grounded in their family relationship of being a parent of the parents.
- Many grandparents put their own grief second and focus on helping and supporting grieving parents.
- Each grandparent's loss is unique, according the meanings that their grandchild's life and death holds for them.
- Individual grandparents have differing ways of coping and making sense of the death of their grandchild.
- Many parents value the role of grandparents in remembering and talking about their dead grandchild.
- Bereaved grandparents are often overlooked or 'forgotten' in existing bereavement care after the sudden death of a child.

REFERENCES

Barranti C 1985 The grandparent–grandchild relationship: family resources in an era of voluntary bonds. Family Relations 34: 343–352

DeFrain J, Jakub D, Mendoza B 1991–2 The psychological effects of sudden infant death on grandmothers and grandfathers. OMEGA, Journal of Death and Dying 24: 165–182

Donnelly KF, Haimes J 1993 Grandparents: overlooked grievers. Thanatos 18: 26–29

Field D 2000 Mortality. Older people's attitudes towards death in England. Mortality 5: 277–297

Fitzgerald M 2001 Grandparent parents. Intergenerational surrogate parenting. Journal of Holistic Nursing 19: 297–307

Fry PS 1997 Grandparents' reactions to the death of a grandchild: an exploratory factor analytic study. OMEGA, Journal of Death and Dying 35: 119–140

Gerner M 1988 To bereaved grandparents. Thanatos 13: 28

Gerner M 1990 For bereaved grandparents. Centering Corporation, Omaha, NE

Gyulay J 1975 The forgotten grievers. American Journal of Nursing 75: 1476–1479

Hurme H 1991 Dimensions of the grandparent role in Finland. In: Smith P (ed) The psychology of grandparenthood. Routledge, London, p 19–31

Jordan J, Kraus D, Ware E 1993 Observations on loss and family development. Family Process 32: 425–440

Kolf J 1995 Grandma's tears. Baker Books, Grand Rapids, MI

Leininger L, Ilse S 1985 Grieving grandparents. Pregnancy and Infant Loss Center, Wayzata, MN

McClowry S, Davies E, May K et al 1987 The empty space phenomenon. Death Studies 11: 361–374

Moss M, Moss S 1997 The impact of family death on older people. New Zealand National Association for Loss and Grief 16: 4,11

Ponzetti J 1992 Bereaved families: a comparison of parents and grandparents' reactions to the death of a child. OMEGA, Journal of Death and Dying 25: 63–71

Ponzetti J, Johnson M 1991 The forgotten grievers: grandparents' reactions to the death of grandchildren. Death Studies 15: 157–167

Rando 1986 The unique issues and impact of the death of a child. In: Rando T (ed) Parental loss of a child. Research Press Company, Champaign, ILL, p 3–44

Riches G, Dawson P 1998 Lost children, living memories: the role of photographs in processes of grief and adjustment among bereaved parents. Death Studies 22: 121–140

Smith P (ed) 1991 The psychology of grandparenthood: an international perspective. Routledge, London

Stewart A 2000 When an infant grandchild dies: family matters. PhD thesis, School of Nursing, University of Wellington, Wellington NZ

Stroebe M, Schut H 2001 Meaning making in the dual process of coping with bereavement. In: Neimeyer R (ed) Meaning reconstruction and the experience of loss. American Psychological Association, Washington, DC, p 55–75

USEFUL SOURCES FOR NURSES AND MIDWIVES

Ponzetti J, Johnson M 1991 The forgotten grievers: grandparents' reactions to the death of grandchildren. Death Studies 15: 157–167

Professional practice and care of bereaved families

The challenge facing many health professionals is how to work with bereaved families. In particular, how to integrate the differing perspectives of grief presented in Section 1 with the different experiences of individuals described in Section 2.

The chapters in this section explore considerations for practice at the time of death and in follow-up bereavement care. The central point is in recognising that people may grieve in different ways and that considerations for practice will require adaptation to suit different people and situations.

The privilege of being allowed into the private world of distressed family members is often balanced by the burden that this may bring. How do health professionals live with stress and loss that they encounter in their practice? How can the ideas in the preceding chapters assist them to identify resources for themselves? This is the focus of the last chapter in the book.

Working in professional practice with bereaved families

> *We shall not cease from exploration*
> *And the end of all our exploring*
> *Will be to arrive where we started*
> *And know the place for the first time*
>
> Eliot 1952

INTRODUCTION

The previous chapters have identified the pain, complexity and uniqueness of grief experienced by different family members following the sudden death of a child. This chapter positions the nurse or midwife in the picture, explores the challenges they face and discusses considerations for their practice. These underpin the next two chapters. Chapter 7 explores working with families around the time of death when midwives and nurses working in accident and emergency, neonatal/paediatric intensive care units and ward settings may be involved. Chapter 8 discusses follow-up care with bereaved families, generally undertaken by professionals working in the community such as health visitors, midwives and practice nurses.

WHY IS WORKING WITH BEREAVED FAMILIES CHALLENGING?

One health visitor wrote, '*I think supporting parents who have lost a child is one of the hardest jobs that a health visitor is expected to do and one which we are hugely ill-prepared and consequently dread.*' Similarly, Gardner (1999) identified that midwives and nurses in the USA, England and Japan felt that they lacked experience, knowledge and confidence when working with families who had experienced a perinatal death. Compassion, concern and a desire to help are some of the feelings that nurses and midwives describe when hearing about the sudden death of a child. Yet the reality of caring for bereaved family members can cause discomfort and even distress. This can arise from interwoven challenges, which can be professional, personal and organisational.

PERSONAL CHALLENGES

It is important to remember and acknowledge that health professionals are firstly people with their own losses, experiences and beliefs. Working with bereaved families can present a personal challenge to oneself as a person for a range of reasons (Worden 1991, pp. 133–134):

- it can be a reminder of the death of oneself and others
- it can trigger a review of spirituality and beliefs about the world and the nature of being
- it can be a reminder of feared pending losses.

Such thoughts and feelings can be heightened at different times in a health professional's life according to personal and professional circumstances.

PROFESSIONAL CHALLENGES

Lack of experience when working with families after sudden child death can be a professional challenge. Dent et al (1996) found that less than half of 186 health visitors in England and Wales had experienced the sudden death of a child in their practice. In addition, there may be a limited number of experienced health professionals available to support and mentor colleagues who may be working with bereaved families for the first time. Even when health professionals have experience of working with families, they may still lack confidence. For some, this can stem from uncertainty about how to respond to some of the reactions of bereaved family members, such as anger, withdrawal and denial (Wright 1996). As one midwife with 15 years experience in practice said, '*I always feel it is a challenge that is outside my comfort zone ... I wonder each time what to do and say when someone cries*'. Many nurses and midwives comment that there was little bereavement content in their preregistration course, any knowledge being gleaned from other colleagues, personal experience and from reading materials. This means that many health professionals want opportunities to support and advance their practice. Provision of such opportunities is partly a reflection of the surrounding organisational culture. Is there support to enable health professionals to talk about their experiences with colleagues, attend clinical supervision sessions or enrol in education workshops? We explore some of these issues further in Chapter 9.

ORGANISATIONAL CHALLENGES

The third challenge facing professionals is the organisational view of bereavement support, both within the health service and in workplace settings. The focus on quality assurance and clinical audit is providing a process to develop standards for care. For example, the Paediatric Intensive Care Society (2002) *Standards for bereavement care* identifies both provision of care for families and the resources, such as education and support, needed by health professionals to be able to provide such care. As standards become integrated into services, it is likely that bereavement care will be seen as a means to sustain the physical, emotional, social and spiritual well-being of family members within the hospital setting.

However, provision of support for families in the community in the months after death is less clear. Comments from some families in England and Wales indicate a perceived lack of support and follow-up after miscarriage (Moulder 2001) and sudden child death (Dent et al 1996). Stories told by some families at mutual help groups reinforce the view that care can be extensive and excellent, or it may be absent. This suggests that provision of care in the past has relied on the interest and commitment of individual health professionals. We hope that development of bereavement care standards will help to address this situation. For example, the London Bereavement Network (www.bereavement.org.uk) was one of the leading organisations in the initiative to develop the *2001 Standards for Bereavement Care: UK Project*. A preliminary version is available from the website and identifies areas where standards are needed to provide effective and safe bereavement care. Until national standards are developed and endorsed, primary care trusts may not see bereavement support as an important part of a community health professional's role, particularly when there are high case loads in both rural and densely populated urban areas. The International Working Group on Death, Dying and Bereavement (cited in Fulton & Bendiksen 1994, p. 420) suggested that, '*Bereavement care should be delivered as effectively and economically as possible and that all persons should have bereavement support readily available*'. Provision of such a service is a form of preventive health care to minimise the detrimental effects that grief can have on the individual's well-being. Comments from parents in Chapter 3 illustrate that many want support from community professionals. Therefore, we urge nurses, midwives and managers of primary health care trusts to view bereavement support as an important part of primary health care.

Having identified some of the challenges facing health professionals, what information and skills can assist them to work confidently with bereaved families?

WHAT IS THE EVIDENCE TO INFORM BEREAVEMENT CARE?

Chapters 3–5 explored the enormity and individuality of grief for family members after the sudden death of a child. In these circumstances, what difference can nurses or midwives make? What form should any intervention take? This section reviews some of the available evidence to inform practice. Where possible, we have cited material relevant to 'sudden' death, but note that some studies of parental bereavement include situations where the death was not sudden. Given the space constraints, we have used parental bereavement as an example and have not reviewed material on interventions with siblings. In addition, we note there is an absence of such material relating to other family members.

Earlier chapters have explored the stressful effects that sudden death of a child can have on parents, siblings and grandparents. Several writers have identified negative cognitive, physical and psychosocial outcomes for family members following the death of a child (e.g. Dyregrov & Mathiesen 1987, Hazzard, Weston & Gutteres 1992, Vance et al 1995). The role of therapists and/or health professionals in parents' experiences of bereavement has been illustrated with examples from clinical practice (see contributors in Raphael 1984, Rando 1986), descriptive data (e.g. Finlay & Dallimore 1991) and stories of bereaved parents (e.g. Hill 1989, Moulder 2001, Radestad 2000). Such information indicates ways in which nurses and midwives might work with bereaved family members. However, which form of bereavement care is best? Who decides if such care is beneficial?

INTERVENTIONS AND OUTCOMES

One of the difficulties facing practitioners seeking evidence to inform practice is the lack of comparability between studies. For example, in a Cochrane review of perinatal death (most substantive update in 1998, further material sought and not found in October 2001) Chambers and Chan (2002, p. 1) identified the **inadequacy** of existing research in terms of methodology, such as small sample size, loss of participants to follow-up and variation between study interventions. They concluded '*that [for women/families after perinatal death] no information is available from randomised trials to indicate whether there is, or is not a benefit from providing specific psychological support or counselling*'. A particular difficulty for the professional who wants to plan bereavement care is the varying forms of intervention, some of which are located within unique contexts of practice that include specialist practitioners or support services. For example, interventions after the sudden death of a child have included structured health visitor support (Dent 2000), group meetings (Murphy 2000) and information materials combined with grief worker visits (Murray et al 2000). Outcome measures vary across studies from standardised scales of physical and mental well-being to reports of parental satisfaction. This raises the debate about what constitutes a beneficial outcome for the provision, and costs, of bereavement care. Furthermore, who decides what is beneficial? In addition, there are differences between studies in the nature of the bereavement event and relationship with the deceased. Some studies include bereaved mothers and fathers (e.g Dent 2000, Murray et al 2000) and others have included the mother (Hughes et al 2002). The bereavement event may range from sudden infant death syndrome (SIDS) to accidents (e.g. Dent 2000) or focus on stillbirths (Hughes et al 2002). The age at which the child died may be at birth (Hughes et al 2002) or older, 12–28 years (Murphy et al 1999). The comments from parents in Chapter 3 illustrated that the meaning of bereavement may vary according to gender, relationship with the deceased and bereavement event. This may account for the observation that an intervention may assist some bereaved people more than others. For example, both Murphy (2000) and Murray et al (2000) reported that an intervention had most effect for bereaved parents who had higher levels of initial distress or were assessed as 'high risk'. This would support Parkes' (2001) premise that many people manage to grieve with the support of family and others without interventions from professionals. This view was reaffirmed in a review of work presented in the recent *Handbook of bereavement research*, which concluded *'counselling and therapy are only needed and effective for a minority of high-risk bereaved people'* (Stroebe et al 2001, p. 761).

The considerable variation in the type of intervention, bereavement event and outcome measures hampers conclusions about bereavement care and indicates that no intervention can be assumed to be beneficial to **all** individuals. This point was supported by Schut et al (2001, p. 706), who concluded from a review of bereavement interventions in general that *'The differences between studies are huge, making detailed comparison hazardous if not impossible'*. This conclusion is congruent with the ideas discussed in Chapter 2, which emphasise different perspectives of grieving. Hence, there remains a need for further, well-designed research using different forms of intervention to identify *'who needs what when'* (Murphy 2000, p. 598). For example, Welch and Bergen (1999–2000) noted that there is no care specifically designed for bereaved adolescent mothers, who are facing bereavement alongside developmental changes with their transition to adulthood.

In addition, many of the available studies relate to counselling and therapy and do not reflect the contexts where nurses and midwives care for bereaved family members. There is a need for research located within nursing and midwifery practice to explore ways in which care might be provided to particular groups of people. In Chapter 2, we cited some examples of innovative research undertaken by nurses and midwives; we hope that there will be an increase in evaluation studies of bereavement care. Meanwhile, current research can help to identify considerations for practice. Some studies offer information that is applicable to practice with particular bereaved individuals after a specific bereavement event with a stated form of care. Nurses and midwives need to search regularly for research studies that are relevant to their scope of practice. Once such information is located, it needs to be critically appraised for methodological validity and clinical applicability using trigger questions offered in texts such as Brown (1999).

THE EFFECT OF CARE

While there is a need for further research, it is also important to consider whether existing forms of bereavement care might cause distress. In the Cochrane review of care following perinatal death, Chambers and Chan (2002, p. 1) noted that current practice focuses on the *'provision of an empathetic, caring environment and strategies to enable the mother and family to accept the reality of death'*. In recent years, this has included encouraging parents to see and hold their child, which Leon (1992, p. 368) described as *'idealization of contact with the dead baby'*. However, are such practices helpful? Radestad et al (1996) undertook a nationwide study in Sweden comparing 380 women who experienced a stillbirth with 379 controls whose child was liveborn. The authors concluded (p. 1507) that, *'staff should not force the mother to hold, caress or kiss the dead child. Such actions were not beneficial in terms of reduced risk for anxiety or depression'*. Hughes et al (2002) reported similar conclusions from a UK study comparing 65 women recruited in the pregnancy after stillbirth with 60 matched controls. The authors noted (p. 114), *'Women who had held their stillborn infant were more depressed than those who only saw the infant, while those who did not see the infant were least likely to be depressed'*. There were similar findings for outcome measures of anxiety and symptoms of post-traumatic stress disorder. Their interpretation was, *'Our findings do not support good-practice guidelines, which state that failure to see and hold the dead child could have adverse effects on parents' mourning'* (Hughes et al 2002, p. 114). By including this material, our intent is not to propose that these conclusions are applied to bereavement care with **all parents**. Rather, it highlights the need to undertake a critical appraisal of such studies to consider **why** these findings may have occurred in these **particular** groups of women studied at this **particular** time point in their grief. As Leon (1992) proposed, there is a need to understand why seeing their dead child might be helpful for some parents and not for others. Careful critical appraisal can then assist nurses and midwives to decide whether the findings are methodologically valid and clinically applicable to the families with whom they work.

The conclusions of Radestad et al (1996) and Hughes et al (2002) caution against practice that prescriptively requires all mothers to have the same care. Does this happen in clinical practice? In a study of neonatal death, Lundqvist and Nilstun (1998, p. 246) found that 60% of 144 Swedish nurses working in neonatal wards *'were of the opinion that the parents' mourning-process is always facilitated when they touch or hold their dead baby'*. Many nurses (74%) had experience of parents refusing to touch or hold their dead baby. Of these nurses, more than half had tried to change the parents' decision through persuasion or other strategies. Rationales for such actions included the belief that the activity would benefit the parents. It is more than 5 years since this study and practice may have changed. However, it is possible that such beliefs and practices exist amongst some health professionals in other countries. Therefore, we believe it is critical for nurses and midwives to question their practice, appraise current research and seek to identify the ways in which certain **forms** of care may suit **different** people at **different** times. This requires nurses and midwives to use their skills to offer choices without necessarily making practice prescriptive.

CONSIDERATIONS FOR PRACTICE

Current practice, including the ideas presented in this book, is a combination of interpretations of available research, comments from motivated groups of family members, and the experience of clinicians. Consequently, we have not presented statements of 'good' or 'best' practice because both terms are value judgements determined by the criteria used and the person undertaking such an interpretation. Instead we have used the term **considerations for practice**, which may require adaptation to suit different bereaved family members. These ideas are based on our experience in practice, listening to family members and existing research. We have grouped the discussion into three main sections offering strategies and skills to address some of the challenges described at the beginning of this chapter:

- recognising diversity in bereavement and grief
- defining professional practice with bereaved families
- working in professional practice with bereaved families.

RECOGNISING DIVERSITY IN BEREAVEMENT AND GRIEF

We believe the material in this book highlights that there are both common threads and unique aspects to people's experiences of bereavement. There are different ways to describe and conceptualise grief. Recognition of diversity is central to practice. Riches and Dawson (2000) used the image of a 'map' to illustrate practice with the complex, individual experience of grief. Each perspective of grief described in Chapter 2 or developed from personal experience, offers a map. The map for each person will be different and may not be the same as that of the health professional offering bereavement care. Riches and Dawson (2000, p. 184) described this:

> ... some of the landscape the bereaved parent or sibling inhabits may seem familiar to us, and we may **think** the maps we already possess might help in guiding them through this territory. But it is **their** journey, not ours, that has to be travelled. Their social and cultural context directly affects their capacity to express or explore their bereavement with others – and with us.

To be able to work with different 'maps' and accommodate different people's experiences requires knowing oneself.

Knowing oneself

Health professionals are individuals, members of families and have their own beliefs, experiences and cultural identity. Such experiences may influence practice and shape the care that is offered to bereaved families. Equally, as we explore in Chapter 9, experiences in practice may cause stress and bereavement to health professionals. We believe that all health professionals working with bereaved family members need to re-view the ways in which personal beliefs about grief and experiences of death can both influence practice and make oneself vulnerable. Such reflection can identify sources of personal challenge (described on p. 110). (For further questions and discussion regarding responses, see Wright 1996, pp. 94–100). Before reading further, take a moment to consider the following questions:

- When did you first experience death?
- How did it affect you?
- How do you feel when you think about dying?
- Are there situations where death makes you uncomfortable?
- Have you made a will?

Knowledge of oneself also includes re-viewing beliefs and experiences as an individual who belongs to various cultures within society, such as being a member of a family or gender group. One perspective of this is 'culturally safe practice', whereby a health professional undertakes '*a process of reflection on his or her own cultural identity and will recognise the impact that (his or her) personal culture has on (his or her) professional practice*' (Nursing Council of New Zealand 2002, p. 7). Recognition of self as different from others enables health professionals to develop professional practice that is sensitive to the beliefs and practices of others. It can also mean recognising that particular behaviours and forms of care may not always be appropriate, or required, by people who identify with a particular religious or ethnic group. As we discussed in Chapter 2, there may be variation within such groups, as well as between groups (see Gunaratnam 1997). Therefore, nurses and midwives might ask individuals whether they would like a particular form of care. This might involve people such as health professionals, spiritual advisors or community leaders. For individuals whose first language is not English, it may require involving interpreters to find out what they would like. To honour diversity also requires having, and demonstrating, respect for individuals and families.

Respect for bereaved families

Respect for people is reflected in the ways in which nurses and midwives provide care and **talk with**, as opposed to **talk at**, bereaved family members. Examples include the following:

- listening to an individual's experience without judging or prescribing the nature of it
- recognising the uniqueness of grief; hence, it may not be appropriate to say 'I know how you feel'
- avoiding platitudes, which may minimise a person's experience
- **never assuming** what a family may wish to do
- offering choices to family members, which may help them to gain a sense of control within the situation
- affirming the identity of the child by naming them, such as '[name] died of cot death, which is also called sudden infant death syndrome or SIDS'

- caring for the dead child with the same respect that would be shown to a living child, which includes the ways that the child is held, touched or talked about.
- affirming the parents' role as guardians of their child, for example 'would you like me to dress [name]?'
- listening, and responding to the language the family members use to describe the death; for example, they may talk about a 'crash' rather than an 'accident' or a 'baby' not a 'fetus'.

DEFINING PROFESSIONAL PRACTICE WITH BEREAVED FAMILIES

Some of the professional and organisational challenges discussed on page 111 relate to defining professional practice. Being able to work confidently with different family members includes the following considerations for practice:

- recognising own competence
- differentiating own professional role
- identifying goal(s) and focus of practice with bereaved families.

Competence to practise

Sometimes nurses and midwives forget that they are well prepared to work with bereaved families. First, they are health professionals registered with a regulatory body, such as the Nursing and Midwifery Council. This registration means that they have met the competencies to practice requiring skills such as professional judgement, assessment and ability to develop appropriate relationships with clients. These are fundamental skills to working with bereaved family members. Second, each nurse or midwife has beliefs and values guiding the way they care for people in their practice. For example, **respect** for the individual is central to the practice of health professionals and is integrated into professional codes of conduct (Nursing and Midwifery Council 2002). Many health professionals have a framework for practice that is located with specific theoretical underpinnings. For example, some midwives use a partnership model of working with women and their families (Guilliland & Pairman 1995) and some nurses use a model of health-promoting practice with families (Hartrick, Lindsey & Hills 1994). Both codes of conduct and frameworks for practice can assist nurses and midwives to work confidently with bereaved people. In addition, nurses and midwives have roles and responsibilities determined by their scope of practice. In some situations, such as being a newly registered practitioner, nurses and midwives may identify that they need support to provide adequate bereavement care to family members. In Chapter 8 we discuss the health professional's responsibility to recognise boundaries of safe and competent practice and to ask for additional support such as a mentor when necessary.

Identifying and differentiating roles in practice

Midwives and nurses have defined roles and responsibilities, which may differ in purpose and nature from other professionals involved in bereavement care. For example, Warland (2000) stated that midwives working with bereaved families are not counsellors. We would agree; it equally applies to nurses. However, nurses and midwives do offer bereavement counselling in the way that Walter (1999, p. xviii) described ' … *they may sit and listen in a highly attentive and disciplined way to what the bereaved have to say*'. So, what is the role that nurses and midwives take with families? Are they 'experts' who can 'treat' or 'fix' the situation? Writing from the context of Australia, Murray (1993) proposed the role of 'companion' for a range of carers, including health professionals, working with families after death of a baby. In this role, companions work '*with families to cope with a normal phenomenon, viz grief. The assumption is that companions help families do something for **themselves** rather than we do something for them*' (Murray 1993, p. 3). This role in bereavement care provides companionship but does not mean being able to 'fix' or 'make' something happen. If this perspective is adopted it affirms the view of Figure 1.1 (p. 4) that nurses and midwives are part of a range of social resources available to bereaved individuals to make sense of their experience. How does clarification of the health professionals' roles help to answer the question that many nurses and midwives ask: 'What am I trying to do with this family?'

The purpose or goal of practice

Sometimes, the obvious is worth reconsidering. Take a moment to consider the following:

- Think about your current experiences with bereaved people.
- What is the goal of your practice when you meet them?
- What is not the goal?.

Some people who attend our workshops reply that they want to 'make it better' for bereaved families. As they recognise, this can present them with a personal and professional challenge because they may be trying to achieve the impossible. Many of the families we have worked with comment that only the return of their live child would 'make it better'. Nurses and midwives cannot achieve this. It can be useful for nurses and midwives to reconsider regularly the purpose of their practice with bereaved family members. The goals in practice need to be congruent with the role and beliefs that a nurse or midwife holds. If a companion role is adopted, then it would not be congruent to 'tell' people how to grieve. Equally, to prescribe a rigid grieving process would not be congruent with a belief in diversity. Based on the material presented in earlier chapters, the purpose of practice might be to promote social, physical, mental and spiritual well-being of family members. The goals in practice might be to:

- assist people to hear the news and recognise that their child is dead
- assist people to find ways to cope with the losses that the death brings
- assist people to find ways to adjust to the reality of a changed world.

A range of resources can assist health professionals to clarify their goal(s) for practice. These include listening to bereaved family members, reflection on practice and appraisal of research and theoretical writings. Recently, frameworks have emerged in the nursing and midwifery literature specifically for working with people experiencing particular bereavement events. For example, Swanson (1999) developed the 'miscarriage model', linked to a theory of caring, and offered an example of using this in practice. Moules (1998) provided a detailed example of working with the beliefs model of Wright, Watson and Bell (1996) to assist a mother who had been told that she was denying her grief after the death of her son. Gordon (1994) described her aims as a bereavement counselling midwifery sister. Riches and Dawson (2000) used interviews with bereaved parents and siblings to identify activities that might be undertaken by any health professional.

Who is the focus of practice?

Part of defining practice is identification of the focus of care. When a child dies suddenly, health professionals' main point of contact is the parents, as Jane described on page 105. This may reflect health service funding contracts that focus available care on the parents or, in some situations, it is determined by practical circumstances where other family members live in distant cities or countries. In 'Setting the scene', we proposed that an important consideration for practice is recognising the ripple of bereavement that extends from the death of one family member. While nurses and midwives may not meet, or be involved in the care of, all the family members, we believe that health professionals need to be **family aware**. Other terms with similar meaning include 'family-centred' or *family-focused*, where *the family context is seen as an important factor in the care of individuals* (Whyte 1997, p. 5). We have used 'aware' to mean remaining alert to, and regardful of, the surrounding family and appreciating that people are not individuals in isolation. Family resources such as the support, beliefs and reactions of other bereaved family members can shape the experience of the bereaved individual. For example, as we described in Chapter 5, some grandparents did not talk about their dead grandchild because they did not know how to reply to the question 'How many grandchildren do you have?' Yet, many parents, such as Pip (p. 104), wanted grandparents to talk about and remember the grandchild. As we discussed in Chapter 1, being aware of the family requires not making assumptions about the structure of the family. Considerations for family awareness in practice could include the following:

- asking parents 'Who is part of your family?'
- offering information and strategies to help parents appreciate and respond to the grief of each other and other family members, and to help other family members appreciate and support parents' grief
- asking parents 'how are [names of other family members] feeling/coping with the death?', thus indicating awareness of the ripple of bereavement that extends from a death
- asking parents about concurrent stresses that may be occurring within the family, such as illness of other family members
- remembering that many families have caregivers, such as nannies, who may have been with the child at the time of death and whose grief may be overlooked.

Having defined the nature of professional practice, the next section explores considerations for working with bereaved family members.

WORKING IN PROFESSIONAL PRACTICE WITH BEREAVED FAMILIES

Working with bereaved people requires maintaining and sustaining professional practice. Considerations include:

- having skills or a 'toolkit' to work with people (e.g. listening, being with, offering choices)
- underpinnings of professional practice (e.g. assessment, confidentiality, maintaining relationships)
- maintaining competency to care for bereaved family members.

In addition, nurses and midwives have a responsibility to sustain themselves when caring for bereaved families, which we discuss further in Chapter 9.

Having a 'toolkit' for practice

Many family members appreciate being listened to, being respected and being offered choices. Nurses and midwives use, and develop, these skills as part of their practice with any individual or family. Some health professionals find it useful to view these as a 'toolkit' for practice with bereaved families. The analogy helps them to visualise the range of skills that they have. Assessment with each individual family member can indicate which 'tool' may be most useful at any particular time. We have identified a range of skills and activities that might be viewed as tools (p. 121). These are framed around the three goals that we proposed on page 118 and make reference to the contexts and resources for grieving (Fig. 1.1, p. 4). We have discussed three possible goals for practice before describing various skills or 'tools':

Assisting family members to hear about and recognise the child's death. Nurses and midwives, like other helpers, act as a '*witness*' (Riches & Dawson 2000, p. 163) to the meanings that family members have about the life and death of their child. Caring activities might focus on the personal and familial resources for grieving and could include acknowledgement, listening, being with family members and assisting them to obtain tokens of remembrance.

Assisting family members to find ways to cope with the losses that the death brings. Death is not just an absence of a physical person or a dreamed-of child in the case of early miscarriage. It brings many losses such as altered everyday activities, body changes for a mother whose milk comes in with no baby to feed, involvement with the criminal justice system following a homicide or changes in family roles for a sibling who now becomes the eldest child. In the hours, days and weeks after a death, nurses and midwives can assist individuals to cope with feelings, thoughts, behaviours, and ill-health that may accompany these losses. Caring activities include those identified in the previous paragraph, which support personal resources to cope. Written and verbal information about other people's perspectives of grief can also provide individuals with new ways to make sense of their experience. Some people who are focused on the pain of their loss may appreciate encouragement to participate in everyday activities such as gardening or going for a walk. From the perspective of the dual process model

(Stroebe & Schut 2001), this could be viewed as helping them move back and forth between loss- and restoration-orientated coping (p. 29). For those who want it, there needs to be the opportunity to talk and have their loss acknowledged. However, as some parents described in Chapter 3, other people may prefer to grieve in private. Many family members appreciate being offered contact details of mutual help groups and other sources of professional assistance.

Assisting family members to find ways to adjust to a new reality.   Nurses and midwives can listen, offer information and support individuals while they find ways of making sense of their changed world. As we noted in Chapter 2, part of the adjustment involves a changed relationship with the dead child. Some family members may want opportunities to sustain a connection with the child. Nurses and midwives can provide such opportunities by asking about symbols, memories or thoughts that link them to the child. As we discussed in Chapter 2, some people may find it difficult to adjust to the new reality and may need additional resources such as a counsellor. We discuss this further in Chapter 8.

Skills and strategies for practice

Nurses and midwives have a range of skills, or tools, to offer assistance to family members. They include:

- acknowledgement
- being with
- listening
- offering time for choices
- offering information
- assisting access to social resources.

Acknowledgement of the child's death

Parents consistently talk about the value of acknowledgement of their grief by others. Many have memories of family, friends and acquaintances who made no acknowledgement of their loss. In such situations, acknowledgement by a nurse or midwife may be critical to legitimise their feelings of grief. It might be as brief as 'I am sorry to hear that your child [name] has died'. Or it may be appropriate to say, 'I don't know what to say'. Nurses and midwives might also consider situations where others may overlook the experience of family members, such as fathers, young siblings or grandparents. Acknowledgement of the loss is also reflected in the physical actions of nurses and midwives, who go to 'be with' the family and provide ongoing support without an expectation that people should 'get over it' within a defined time-period.

Being with bereaved family members

The stories of family members indicate that the value of nurses and midwives 'being with' a bereaved family should not be underestimated. Sometimes, health professionals find it difficult to be with a bereaved person who withdraws into silence or tears. As Wright (1996, p. 72) noted, '*This can be particularly uncomfortable for nurses, whose ethos is about working, caring, or being busy. Nurses have great difficulty in seeing the value of just being there without putting it right. It is not like being able to put a bandage on and "making it better". The wound is deep and painful and the attempt at first-aid appears to produce poor results.'* However, being silent with bereaved people can have a purpose; it allows the person to withdraw into their thoughts, or to just 'be' exhausted. The nature of 'being with' is about human companionship during a time when people are grappling to understand their changed world. Being with someone may include just sitting in the same place or it might involve physical touch; this depends on whether the person and the health professional are comfortable with such contact.

Listening

Not everyone wants to talk with a health professional whether known or unknown. However, many family members appreciate the opportunity to have someone listen to them with complete attention. Nurses and midwives have the skills to offer this to bereaved family members. In a study of mothers bereaved of a child aged from birth to 14 months, Farnsworth and Allen (1996, p. 366) noted that ' *... nurses were frequently mentioned by mothers as good listeners who were helpful to them in beginning to understand grieving as a unique process'*. Listening may enable the bereaved person to talk and thus help them to:

- make the loss 'real'
- describe and 'off-load' feelings
- gain new insights for self through description to another person
- receive acknowledgement for the loss.

As we noted in 'Setting the scene', the opportunity to tell their stories may help family members to gain new insights (Walter 1996) and to link their sense of past, present and future into a revised life-story (White & Epston 1990). While nurses and midwives are not narrative therapists, they are familiar with stories as part of working with clients to make meaning of their health experiences. Some family members appreciate being encouraged to tell their stories of the child's death. Questions that may offer the opportunity to tell a story include:

- tell me about [name]
- what happened when [name] died?
- how do you feel about [name]?
- what are the things that you remember about [name]?

Our experience with bereaved family members indicates that as people gain new insights and knowledge, their story may change. Therefore, nurses and midwives need to consider that stories are told from different perspectives, to different audiences, at different times. Frank (1995, p. 159) writing from the context of illness proposed that the challenge for any health professional is to 'truly listen to others' stories'. This requires engaging with the person's experience and avoiding the imposition of interpretations based on the health professional's world view. Otherwise, as Braun and Berg (1994, p. 126) suggested, '*Providing explanations or advice that*

**Box 6.1
Guidelines for
befrienders**

You are listening when ...

- You come quietly into my private world and let me be me.
- You really try to understand me when I do not make much sense.
- You hold back your desire to give me good advice.
- You don't take my problem from me but trust me to deal with it in my own way.
- You give me enough room to discover for myself why I feel upset, and enough time to think for myself what is best.
- You allow me the dignity of making my own decisions even though you feel I am wrong.

From the Foundation for the Study of Infant Deaths (2000, p. 8).
(with permission of FSID, UK, www.sids.org.uk/fsid)

does not correspond with the parents' views of the experience is likely to cause anger and frustration'. Instead, it may be possible to listen and sometimes offer suggestions by using the phrase 'I wonder if ...'. Box 6.1 is an excerpt from the *Guidelines for befrienders* published by the Foundation for the Study of Infant Deaths; it offers one perspective of being listened to without being imposed upon.

Offering time to make choices

Interspersed with listening and being with bereaved family members is offering choices and information. Throughout this text, we have suggested that health professionals consider offering choices to family members rather than making assumptions about what 'should' be part of their experience. Where possible, nurses and midwives can encourage family members to take time to make decisions about available options. In Chapter 7, we discuss choices such as having a photograph or choosing to see their dead child as ones that are not 'once-only' options. Family members, and in particular parents, can take several hours or days to decide what they want to do. Clearly, such choices have to be made before burial or cremation, but many choices do not need to be a rushed decision. Written and verbal information can assist families to make choices.

Offering information to family members

Many family members want information. It can provide new insights, coping strategies and knowledge about what is happening. Nurses and midwives can share information with family members as part of conversations. Information also exists in written or visual form including leaflets, books, websites and videos (Appendices 1–6). In particular, parents may need resources to help them support bereaved siblings (Appendices 2, 4, 6, 7).

We have emphasised throughout this book our belief that nurses and midwives should critically appraise the ideas that inform their practice. Such appraisal equally applies to written or visual information that might be recommended to family members. Some resources present a particular perspective of grief, such as stages of grieving or the need to express grief through talking and crying. Some people may not find these ideas helpful; others will read the information they want and ignore the remaining content. A few may even feel '*grief guilt*' (Miles & Demi 1986, p. 107) based on a view that their behaviour does not meet personal or societal expectations of grieving. Therefore, we believe, nurses and midwives need to consider what they are recommending, indicating to family members that different resources suit different people.

In the appendices we have included lists of resources. Some have an explanatory comment where we have found an item useful in some situations. Resources are constantly changing and a useful strategy in any practice setting is to have a designated person establish and maintain a current resource file of materials for colleagues to use with bereaved families.

Assisting family members to access social resources

The sudden death of a child presents a huge challenge to family members. Support from other people is a social resource that can help to buffer the stressful effects of bereavement (Cohen & Wills 1985, Kessler, Price & Wortman 1985). It may be forthcoming from other family members (who are also bereaved) or from friends, work colleagues, mutual help groups, religious advisers, and practitioners such as midwives, nurses, doctors, social workers, counsellors and therapists.

Family, friends and others. The comments from bereaved family members presented earlier in the book, illustrate that many bereaved people want and appreciate the support of others. The comments in Chapters 3–5 illustrate that many people receive and give support within the family. However, discomfort and uncertainty may cause potential supporters to stay away or they may be unable to communicate in a helpful way (Lehman et al 1986). Sometimes, nurses and midwives may be able to assist would-be supporters by offering suggestions about how to help bereaved family members. Many mutual help groups and self-help texts (Appendices 1 and 5) provide written suggestions for friends and work colleagues, which include cooking a meal, caring for the children, ringing up the funeral director, remembering anniversaries, asking the parents 'How are you?' For people who may have had little personal experience of bereavement, these can provide the triggers to keep in touch with the bereaved family.

Professional support and non-statutory organisations including mutual help groups. Apart from contact with nurses and midwives; families may receive support from other professionals, such as GP, paediatrician, social worker, teachers at the child's school, counsellor, therapist, psychiatrist and psychologist. The extent and nature of follow-up varies but is often limited by funding and availability of staff. Family members may need assistance from a nurse or midwife to access resources from a range of organisations. However, the existence of other resources does not remove the need for available and ongoing support from health professionals. Organisations such as Foundation for the

Study of Infant Death, The Compassionate Friends, Victim Support and local churches offer 'befrienders' who can listen and offer information. Their volunteers have attended designated workshops and may participate in a process of debriefing or supervision. Some organisations have counsellors, whose services may be free or fee-based. Some people choose to attend group meetings; others may just appreciate reading regular newsletters. Groups exist in different forms from chatrooms on the internet to face-to-face meetings; the latter may include combinations of bereaved families only, structured activities, open discussion, support or facilitation from professionals. Klass (1982) provided a useful discussion on the roles that professionals might take in such groups. In addition, some groups undertake activities such as memorial services, developing information booklets and providing training sessions for health professionals.

REQUIREMENTS OF PROFESSIONAL PRACTICE

Underpinning all the skills (or tools) that nurses and midwives have available to work with bereaved families, are the requirements of professional practice such as assessment, documentation and maintaining competent practice.

ASSESSMENT AND DOCUMENTATION

Assessment forms the basis of planning care. Assessment of the individual family member may include asking about their physical, emotional, spiritual and social well-being. To maintain an awareness of the family context might include asking the individual about their perceptions of the well-being of their family. This may highlight tensions between family members, a need for information about a particular issue or an opportunity to make suggestions such as 'Have you told your daughter how you feel?' The use of assessment tools to guide care is discussed further in Chapter 8. The importance of detailed documentation of observations and of interventions cannot be underestimated as an ongoing record of care and changes over time. In addition, parents whose baby dies around the time of birth may want copies of the documentation as a token of remembrance of their child's life and death.

CONFIDENTIALITY

Under existing legislation in different countries, maintaining confidentiality of information is a central part of practice. This includes having regard for auditory privacy as part of conversations with families, particularly in a hospital setting. Many health care organisations have policies regarding confidentiality; therefore, health professionals need to be aware of these and the relevant legislation with regard to practice with any individual.

MANAGING RELATIONSHIPS WITH FAMILY MEMBERS

'Relationships are the basis of being with' and listening to parents and other family members in the short and long term. Nurses and midwives gain experience in managing boundaries in relationships throughout their daily practice. In the context of bereavement care, occasionally families may reject the support of nurses and midwives. This may not be a personal rejection; it may be because the professional was the bearer of bad news such as 'they told me my child was dead' or because an individual finds it difficult to be 'in need' of support (Stewart 1988). In contrast, some family members may become overly reliant on the time, resources and support of a health professional. At the beginning of a helping relationship, there is often an element of dependency because a bereaved person may need and want support. However, over weeks and months, this generally diminishes as the person grieves and adjusts to a different life.

Assessment may help the nurse or midwife to anticipate and minimise the likelihood of overdependence. Indicators may include:

- social isolation and the absence of support from family or friends
- preference to see one health professional to the point of rejecting others
- a strong interest in the personal life of the health professional
- a rejection of suggestions that follow-up bereavement contact will end.

Strategies to minimise such dependence can include:

- having a clearly stated contract of care so that both the family member and health professional have realistic expectations of care, which includes the understanding that bereavement care does not continue indefinitely
- clarifying with the family members any perceptions of dependence, 'I wonder if you are wanting me to fix it for you?'
- suggesting the need for involvement of other support resources (e.g. counsellor, family, mutual help group)
- using professional supervision to explore strategies that can be used in the situation.

MAINTAINING COMPETENCY TO PRACTICE

Maintaining skills and knowledge is central to competent practice as a nurse or midwife. This can include reflection and professional supervision, which are discussed in Chapter 9. It also includes maintaining currency of knowledge and developing skills. Nurses and midwives need to keep informed about issues relevant to practice with bereaved families. This can include:

- sourcing information from current journals about the topics of bereavement, child death and particular bereaved groups relevant to scope of practice
- accessing resources and information to develop personal practice (Appendix 8)
- reading stories written by bereaved family members to gain insights into their realities
- maintaining awareness of changes in (a) legislation regarding age of viability and (b) local practices such as the storage of children's bodies while awaiting a postmortem
- attending a mutual help group to meet with bereaved families
- talking with other health professionals who have expertise and/or specific knowledge that will inform own practice
- accessing education workshops, courses and conferences to gain further knowledge for practice.

The earlier discussion about the challenges facing health professionals highlights that this can be a very demanding and humbling area of practice, not least because death and grief are part of life and yet defy a universal understanding. Riches and Dawson (2000, p. 83) encouraged professionals to cope with the challenges:

> the ability to feel 'comfortable' with uncertainty, to accept limitations both to personal knowledge and to the capacity to help or put things right and a willingness to keep learning – especially from bereaved people themselves – are central to professional practice in a postmodern world.

This view reaffirms our comment in 'Setting the scene' that no single text will provide definitive answers for practice. Instead, nurses and midwives can assess their own personal resources, identify their learning needs and then identify a strategy to meet those needs. The current emphasis on reflective practice supports this approach and we would encourage everyone to undertake a self-assessment of their practice. This can form the basis of a proposed plan for professional development and could be included in a professional portfolio of practice. Before reading further, take a moment to answer the following questions:

- What do you feel are your strengths when working with bereaved people/ families?
- What skills would you like to develop in your work with bereaved people/ families?
- What are the resources that you need to to develop these skills?

Part of maintaining professional practice also includes consideration of the surrounding work environment. On page 111 we identified organisational issues that may challenge health professionals working with bereaved families. Nurses and midwives can take a proactive role to identify areas in existing services that might be reviewed. This might include participation in audits and consultation with other health professionals and consumers to identify strategies to enhance bereavement care. For example, the Paediatric Intensive Care Society (2002) includes an example tool for bereavement audit. Areas that might be reviewed in any clinical setting include:

- having staffing and skill mix to enable staff to spend sufficient time with families
- identifying whether support and follow-up is available to families who experience death of a child from miscarriage through to teenage years
- establishing mentoring and information-sharing practices in the workplace
- developing the role of a key-worker to liaise between agencies involved with families.

SUMMARY

This chapter has set the scene of professional practice with bereaved families. We have strongly emphasised in this book that bereaved family members have a range of resources to cope with, and make sense of, their experience. Similarly, nurses and midwives are well equipped; they have many resources and skills to work confidently with bereaved families. In the following chapters, we explore specific considerations for practice when working with families at the time of their child's death and then over subsequent months.

SUMMARY POINTS

- Nurses and midwives face a number of challenges when working with bereaved families.
- Confidence to work with bereaved families includes defining professional practice, such as the role and purpose of working with families.
- Various considerations for practice have been derived from comments from families, research and clinical experience. They remain as considerations to be interpreted and adapted to suit different individuals and situations.
- Skills that nurses and midwives bring to their work with bereaved families include acknowledgement of the death, being with and listening to family members, offering choices and information, and assisting family members to access resources.
- Health professionals are one social resource that can assist bereaved family members. Other resources include family, friends, mutual help groups and non-statutory bereavement agencies.

REFERENCES

Braun M, Berg D 1994 Meaning reconstruction in the experience of parental bereavement. Death Studies 18: 105–129

Brown S 1999 Knowledge for health care practice. W B Saunders, Philadelphia, PA

Chambers H, Chan FY 2002 Support for women/families after perinatal death (Cochrane Review). In: The Cochrane Library Issue 1. Update Software, Oxford

Cohen S, Wills TA 1985 Stress, social support, and the buffering hypothesis. Psychological Bulletin 98: 301–357

Dent A 2000 Support for families whose child dies suddenly from accident or illness. PhD thesis, School of Policy Studies, University of Bristol, UK

Dent A 2002 Family support after sudden child death. Community Practitioner 75: 469–473

Dent A, Condon L, Fleming P et al 1996 A study of bereavement care after sudden and unexpected death. Archives of Disease in Childhood 74: 522–526

Dyregrov A, Mathiesen SB 1987 Similarities and differences in mothers' and fathers' grief following the death of an infant. Scandinavian Journal of Psychology 28: 1–15

Eliot T 1952 Four quartets. The complete poems and plays of TS Eliot. Harcourt Brace, New York

Farnsworth E, Allen K 1996 Mothers' bereavement. Experiences of marginalization, stories of change. Family Relations 45: 360–367

Finlay I, Dallimore D 1991 Your child is dead. British Medical Journal 302: 1524–1525

Foundation for Sudden Infant Death. Guidelines for befrienders. Foundation for Sudden Infant Death, London

Frank A 1995 The wounded storyteller. University of Chicago Press, Chicago, IL

Fulton R, Bendiksen R 1994 Death and identity. Charles Press, Philadelphia, PA

Gardner JM 1999 Perinatal death: uncovering the needs of midwives and nurses and exploring helpful interventions in the United States, England and Japan. Journal of Transcultural Nursing 10: 120–130

Gordon M 1994 Bereavement counselling: a full-time job. Modern Midwife 4: 27–28

Guilliland K, Pairman S 1995 The midwifery partnership: a model for practice (Monograph 1). Department of Nursing and Midwifery, Victoria University, Wellington, NZ

Gunaratnam Y 1997 Culture is not enough: a critique of multi-culturalism in palliative care. In: Field D, Hockey J, Small N (eds) Death, gender and ethnicity. Routledge, London, p 166–186

Hartrick G, Lindsey A, Hills, M 1994 Family nursing assessment: meeting the challenge of health promotion. Journal of Advanced Nursing 20: 85–91

Hazzard A, Weston J, Gutteres C 1992 After a child's death: factors related to parental bereavement. Journal of Development and Behavioural Paediatrics 13: 24–30

Hill S 1989 Family. Penguin, London

Hughes P, Turton P, Hopper E et al 2002 Assessment of guidelines for good practice in psychosocial care of mothers after stillbirth: a cohort study. Lancet 360: 114–118

Kessler R, Price R, Wortman C 1985 Social factors in psychopathology: stress, social support and coping processes. Annual Review of Psychology 36: 531–572

Klass D 1982 Self-help groups for the bereaved: theory, theology and practice. Journal of Religion and Health 21: 307–324

Lehman DR, Ellard JH, Wortman CB 1986 Social support the bereaved: recipients' and providers' perspectives on what is helpful. Journal of Consulting and Clinical Psychology 52: 218–231

Leon I 1992 Perinatal loss: a critique of current hospital practices. Clinical Pediatric 31: 366–374

Lundqvist A, Nilstun T 1998 Neonatal death and parents' grief. Experience, behaviour and attitudes of Swedish nurses. Scandinavian Journal Caring Science 12: 246–250

Miles M, Demi A 1986 Guilt in bereaved parents. In: Rando T (ed) Parental loss of a child. Research Press, Champaign, IL, p 97–118

Moulder C 2001 Miscarriage: women's experiences and needs, 2nd edn. Routledge, London

Moules N 1998 Legitimizing grief: challenging beliefs that constrain practice. Journal of Family Nursing 4: 142–66

Murphy S 2000 The use of research findings in bereavement programs: a case study. Death Studies 24: 285–602

Murphy S, das Gupta A, Cain, K et al 1999 Changes in parents' mental distress after the violent death of an adolescent or young adult child: a longitudinal prospective analysis. Death Studies 23: 129–159

Murray J 1993 An ache in their hearts. University of Queensland, Brisbane, Australia

Murray JA, Terry DJ, Vance JC et al 2000 Effects of a program of intervention on parental distress following infant death. Death Studies 24: 275–305

Nursing and Midwifery Council 2002 Code of Professional Conduct. UKCC, London. Available online: http://www.nmc-uk.org, accessed 1 Feb 2003

Nursing Council of New Zealand 2002 Guidelines for cultural safety, the Treaty of Waitangi, and Maori health in nursing and midwifery education and practice. NCNZ, Wellington, NZ

Paediatric Intensive Care Society 2002 Standards for bereavement care. Available from Secretary, Dr C Stack. PICU, Sheffield Children's Hospital, Western Bank, Sheffield S10 2TH, UK

Parkes C 2001 A historical overview of the scientific study of bereavement. In: Stroebe M, Hansson R, Stroebe W et al (eds) Handbook of bereavement research. American Psychological Association, Washington, DC, p 25–45

Radestad I 2000 When a meeting is also farewell. Books for Midwives, Cheshire, UK

Radestad I, Steineck G, Nordin C, Sjogren B 1996 Psychological complications after stillbirth – influence of memories and immediate management: population based study. British Medical Journal 312: 1505–1507

Rando T 1986 The unique issues and impact of the death of a child. In: Rando T (ed) Parental loss of a child. Research Press, Buckingham, UK

Raphael B 1984 The anatomy of bereavement, 3rd edn. Unwin Hyman, London

Riches G, Dawson P 2000 An intimate loneliness: supporting bereaved parents and siblings. Open University Press, Buckingham, UK

Schut H, Stroebe M, van den Bout J et al 2001 The efficacy of bereavement interventions determining who benefits. In: Stroebe M, Hansson R, Stroebe W et al (eds) Handbook of bereavement research. American Psychological Association, Washington, DC, p 705–737

Stewart M 1988 The anguish of being in need. Bereavement Care 7: 17–18

Stroebe M, Schut H 2001 Meaning making in the dual process of coping with bereavement. In: Neimeyer R (ed) Meaning reconstruction and the experience of loss. American Psychological Association, Washington, DC, p 55–75

Stroebe M, Hansson R, Stroebe W et al 2001 Future directions for bereavement research. In: Stroebe M, Hansson R, Stroebe W et al (eds) Handbook of bereavement research. American Psychological Association, Washington, DC, p 741–766

Swanson K 1999 Research-based practice with women who have had miscarriages. IMAGE: Journal of Nursing Scholarship 31: 339–345

Vance J, Boyle F, Najman J et al 1995 Gender differences in parental psychological distress following perinatal death or sudden infant death syndrome. British Journal of Psychiatry 167: 806–811

Walter T 1996 A new model of grief: bereavement and biography. Mortality 1: 7–27

Walter T 1999 On bereavement: the culture of grief. Open University Press, Buckingham, UK

Warland J 2000 The midwife and the bereaved family. Ausmed, Ascot Vale, Australia

Welch K, Bergen M 1999–2000 Adolescent parent mourning reactions associated with stillbirth or neonatal death. OMEGA, Journal of Death and Dying 40: 435–451

White M, Epston D 1990 Narrative means to therapeutic ends. Norton, New York

Whyte D 1997 Family nursing: a systemic approach to nursing work with families. In: Whyte D (ed) Explorations in family nursing. Routledge, London, p 1–26

Worden JW 1991 Grief counselling and grief therapy, 2nd edn. Routledge, London

Wright B 1996 Sudden death, 2nd edn. Churchill livingstone, Edinburgh

Wright LM, Watson W, Bell J 1996 Beliefs. The heart of healing in families and illness. Basic Books, New York

USEFUL SOURCES FOR NURSES AND MIDWIVES

Hindmarch C 2000 On the death of a child 2nd edn. Radcliffe Medical Press, Oxford

Kohner N, Henley A 2001 When a baby dies, 2nd edn. Routledge, London

Moulder C 2001 Miscarriage: women's experiences and needs, 2nd edn. Routledge, London

Riches G, Dawson P 2000 An intimate loneliness: supporting bereaved parents and siblings. Open University Press, Buckingham, UK

Warland J 2000 The midwife and the bereaved family. Ausmed, Ascot Vale, Australia

Wright B 1996 Sudden death, 2nd edn. Churchill Livingstone, London

Supporting bereaved families at the time of death

> See first that you yourself deserve to be a giver, and an instrument of giving.
> For in truth it is life that gives unto life – while you, who deem yourself a giver, are but a witness.
>
> Kahlil Gibran
> *The Prophet*

INTRODUCTION

The sudden death of a child has the potential to render individuals and groups feeling helpless. It is a major life crisis. Parents, bereaved suddenly, may be drained of all power, unable to focus their thoughts and to find a voice. Many parents may not know what is allowed and may be fearful of asking. Does their child still belong to them? Can they still touch and hold their child? What will happen to the body? In addition, they are often faced with telling other family members about the death, including surviving children. So, how can health professionals care for families around the time of death? This chapter explores considerations for nurses and midwives working with bereaved families. Materials that have predominantly focused on sudden death, many of which have been discussed in earlier chapters, inform the content. These include parents' comments, research and our clinical experience. In order to keep the focus on practical considerations, we have only included references to key materials.

In Chapter 6, we used examples to propose that available evidence does not support an assumption that all bereaved families will benefit from or require the same care. In this chapter, we continue to offer considerations for practice that need to be adapted to each situation and individual. This requires nurses and midwives to use their professional judgement and also knowledge of research relevant to the particular group of people with whom they are working. For example, practice needs to be adapted to differing causes of death and different family groups such as single parents, two parents, step-parents, foster parents and grandparents.

TIME BEFORE DEATH

CONTEXT OF PRACTICE

As we noted in Chapter 6, nurses and midwives need to consider both the context to their practice and their goals when working with bereaved families. At the time of death there are a number of considerations related to the context:

- appreciating that the sudden and unexpected nature of the death means that parents and family members may be shocked, disbelieving and confused
- recognising that while parents are the main point of contact at the time of death, the bereavement extends to other family members; support and information offered to the parents may assist other family members' grief
- appreciating concurrent stressors may exist within the family at the time of death that reduce the ability of family members to cope with, or hear, the news that their child has died
- recognising the complexity of blended families; for example, where parents have new partners there may be several family groups needing information and support from health professionals
- appreciating the need for clear communication: where family members have a limited understanding of English, this may require accessing interpreters, spiritual advisors or community leaders to translate information and support families; written information materials may need to be developed to suit the language and culture of ethnic groups in some localities.

Most importantly, care at the time of death lays the foundations for the family over future months and years. The acronym COMPASSION provides reflective questions and pointers as a basis for practice (Box 7.1). Take a moment to look at this before reading further.

Box 7.1 Caring for bereaved families at the time of death: laying the foundations

C are and compassion are key elements. Do you have these qualities?

O ffer yourself as a fellow human being, listening carefully and actively. Remember your body language will convey what you are thinking.

M essage of grief: recognise that the pain of grief cannot be taken away. There are no instant solutions and, therefore, there are no hard and fast rules for how to respond.

P reparation is important. Are you ready to care for bereaved families? Do you know where to find information, equipment and who to contact to offer support?

A ccept the parent(s) reactions. Can you deal with anger or silence?

S eek help if you feel overwhelmed or out of your depth. Who can you go and talk to?

S upervision or workplace support should be available to you. Ensure that you have sufficient time to debrief and learn from each situation.

I nformation is important to parents and family members. Do you know where to find written information for families?

O ffer choices to parent(s) to help them make informed decisions.

N otify other health professionals and agencies, particularly in primary health, so that they can continue the care you have started.

DEATH IN THE HOSPITAL SETTING

Health professionals in the community often make contact with families in the hours and days following the death. However, it is generally hospital staff who have to tell families of their child's death and offer information, which includes material about legal requirements, choices to be with the child, funerals and registration of death. For example, Dent et al (1996) found that of 42 UK families whose child had died suddenly and unexpectedly aged from 1 week to 12 years, half the deaths occurred in a hospital. Of these, over half had died in paediatric intensive care units (PICU), a quarter in accident & emergency departments, 14% in neonatal intensive care units (NICU) and a small percentage on hospital wards. Of the children who had died in the community, as far as could be established, all were taken to the local hospital for further treatment or for verification of death. In addition, many deaths of babies during pregnancy and labour occur in the hospital setting. Although children with life-threatening illness are not included in this book, occasionally, they die suddenly on paediatric wards. Some of the considerations discussed in this chapter may be applicable to their families.

Health professionals' practice at the time of death may well influence families' experiences. Bereaved family members may examine, for weeks, the statements and actions of hospital staff, and the events of the day of death may be replayed for a lifetime (Henrietta & Vanbrunt 1982, Soreff 1984, Korth 1988). This can place a considerable challenge and potential burden on health professionals. However, as Hindmarch (2000, p. 116) noted, the *sincerity of trying to do one's best is what matters*.

As we noted in 'Setting the scene', there are many situations where family members may perceive death as sudden, although the death was not instantaneous. In contrast to how life was before, the death is unexpected and, therefore, sudden. In reality there may be some hours or days before the death during which time health professionals can offer care. For example:

- a child treated for meningitis before dying in PICU
- a baby born prematurely at 24 weeks who dies 36 hours later despite treatment in NICU
- a child maintained on life-support after a road-traffic accident until a decision is made to withdraw support.

In such situations, it is helpful to allocate the care to a specific person, or people, who can be with and provide support for parents at a time of great uncertainty in an unfamiliar environment. Human companionship at such a time may be very important. Regardless of the length of treatment preceding death, parents generally want to be kept informed about what is happening to their child and to be prepared if possible for the eventuality of death (Dent et al 1996). If it becomes apparent from a range of investigations either that death is imminent or that life-support is the only means of continued survival, choices may include continuing care in hospital, being with the child while life-support is withdrawn or taking the dying child home. All choices are enormous decisions that may have lifelong repercussions for families. Sometimes, when a choice is made by parent(s), other family members may not support it. Consequently, ongoing tensions or recriminations may occur. Nurses and midwives can support parents and other family members by listening, answering questions and helping them to think and talk about possible choices. In addition, medical colleagues need to be available to meet family members, answer questions and talk about options.

DEATH AT THE TIME OF DELIVERY OR BIRTH

With miscarriage or stillbirth, parents are faced with the unexpected death of their child at the time of birth. While the parents may have known about the death for several hours or days, the death is often perceived as sudden in that it happened 'out of the blue'. As we discussed in Chapter 2, grief may vary according to the relationship and the circumstances of death. Information to assist parents includes:

- discussion about delivery (e.g. where, how, analgesia)
- possible complications (e.g. an incomplete miscarriage will require an operation under general anaesthetic to remove remaining products of conception)
- their choices to be able to see/hold their baby or, in the case of an early miscarriage, the tissues that form a developing baby.

For further details see Warland (2000). As we noted in Chapter 6, careful consideration needs to be given to language used in such discussions. While 'products of conception' may have a clinically useful meaning for health professionals' communication, it may mean a wanted 'baby' for parents.

A CHILD DYING AT HOME

A child may die at home when born with an unexpected physical condition that leads to death. It may be long remembered by family members, as Rochelle described in her poem at the beginning of Chapter 4. Some families may want to have their child at home but are fearful of being alone with a dying child. The information that parents need to consider includes the following:

- what equipment will accompany the child?
- what skills will the family need to care for the child?
- what support is available from health professionals?
- how quickly are health professionals likely to be able to reach the home when contacted?
- what is likely to happen when the child dies: will it be rapid or lengthy, such as a period of laboured breathing?
- who to contact when the child dies?
- what support is available from family and friends?

WITHDRAWING LIFE-SUPPORT

The decision to withdraw life-support is one that most people hope they will never face. Again parents need information to understand what investigations have been done to indicate that withdrawal of support is a reasonable option. They also need time to reach a decision and to be able to ask questions to assist their decisions. As with resuscitation, health professionals need to consider the presence of the family at the time when equipment is removed. Any exclusion from the moment of their child's death may become the focus of their grief for years to come. Rose, who offered her story in Chapter 3, has remained angry for many years because she wanted the chance to be with Ruby when life-support was turned off.

> *They gave us plenty of time and we went in and we had her blessed before they did it and talked to her and said good-bye. We went and sat in our room. They didn't actually give us the choice to stay there because they said it would be very unpleasant.*

RESUSCITATION

Practice has changed from the time when parents had little access to their child in hospital. Most children's hospitals in the UK now operate open access to parents, which means that they need never be separated from their child. However, attendance of parents during resuscitation varies in different localities. Hindmarch (2000, p. 122) identified that health professionals may object because they believe that:

- *staff feel inhibited*
- *parents need protecting from seeing aggressive treatment*
- *parents get in the way*
- *staff are vulnerable to criticism.*

She noted that the issue is whether the rights of parents to be with their child are respected and a choice offered. Some families will not take the option. Those who do choose are generally focused on the child not the treatment. Or, as Pip described, parents will decide to leave at some point.

> *They worked on her for quite a while but she never really rallied again. For a little while she did do a couple of breaths on her own but that was about it really. After that had been going on for an hour, they were still working on her and we were still in the room, I said to Donald, 'I think I'll go somewhere else now'.*

GIVING THE NEWS OF DEATH

It is often a doctor who tells the parents, and accompanying family members, that their child has died (Dent et al 1996). However, all nurses and midwives need to consider ways in which the news might be imparted. Parents remember the words used and often appreciate the difficulty of the task facing the health professional. While most of the parents in the study by Dent et al (1996) had been told about their child's death in a sensitive manner, this does not always happen. Sarah described what happened 24 hours after Matthew's birth:

> They called us into a side room and told us that he wasn't going to live because his heart wasn't formed properly. I can remember the cardiologist because he was very matter of fact – there was no emotion at all. Whereas the paediatrician was kind and very compassionate. I felt sorry for the cardiologist because I thought, 'He just doesn't know how to cope with this, and he's pretending that it's like a sore thumb or sore toe.'

Von Bloch (1996) discussed various issues pertinent to breaking the news of sudden death. Where possible nurses and midwives might consider that the news of the death should be given:

- by the person involved in caring for the child
- as soon as possible after the death
- to both parents or, if this is not possible, then asking a friend or other family member to come to be with a lone parent
- in a quiet setting that is private and comfortable with access to a telephone, refreshments and toys for any accompanying children
- by using simple, straightforward words such as 'I am sorry to tell you that your child [name] is dead'
- avoiding ambiguous euphemisms such as 'lost'
- avoiding medical terminology such as 'second trimester fetus' to describe the parents' baby who died at 23 weeks of gestation
- allowing enough time for families to assimilate the information that their child is dead and then being available to answer questions subsequently
- showing an appreciation in both words and gestures of the enormity of the loss for the family.

Giving news of the death is the first affirmation that death has actually happened. Because of the enormity of the news, combined with the unexpectedness of a sudden death, shock and disbelief may prevent the reality of the situation from being absorbed. People in shock respond in different ways. Some may withdraw from the situation or deny the death. The facts may need telling at the parents' pace, checking out what has been heard and repeating where necessary. Some parents may become hysterical, wailing, crying, yelling or screaming and pounding their fists. While it is painful to observe, this may be the way they respond when distressed.

Occasionally, angry feelings may be directed at health professionals with accusations of 'failure' to care for the child. In such a situation it can be hard not to feel defensive. One way to diffuse such anger may be to listen to the person without initially defending, or responding to, any of the accusations. The range of ways in which family members respond can create a feeling of helplessness in the health professional (Wright 1996); a sense of 'What **can** I do?' Yet, it is often 'being with' family members and showing compassion that is remembered.

HELPING PARENTS TO TELL CHILDREN THE NEWS

Generally, unless siblings are part of the family group receiving the news, it is parents not health professionals who tell siblings about the death. Health professionals can support parents to do so by indicating the following points to consider:

- giving a clear explanation to children of any age
- using words such as 'died' not euphemisms such as 'lost' or 'went to sleep'
- allowing and respecting a child's reactions
- reassuring the child that that they are loved and perhaps expressing it with a hug
- allowing time for questions
- being prepared that a child's reaction to the news may reflect a need for security, e.g. 'do you still love me?'

Pointers to help parents support bereaved children are provided in Appendix 7.

AFTER HEARING THE NEWS

After being told the news of the child's sudden death, many parents need time to assimilate this information. The physical care of family members should not be overlooked. This means ensuring that they have access to refreshments while they are in a hospital setting. There may be particular requirements for family members. For example, a mother who has recently experienced childbirth may need analgesia and information about suppression of lactation (see Warland 2000). The shock of the unexpected news, combined with the exhaustion and physical pain that can follow, means that all parents need to be reassured that they have time to make choices regarding their child.

Some families will want to go home to a familiar place, possibly to return later. Some parents may be in a state of severe shock after news of the sudden death and need to be cared for. It is worth checking how the parent(s) will get home. Some parents may have come to hospital with their child by ambulance; others may be too shocked to drive. Arranging transport can greatly assist parents and help them to feel nurtured. If a parent has come alone, then nurses or midwives may need to arrange for someone known and trusted to be with them when they return home. In some circumstances where a child has died in a hospital ward, there may be the option for the parents to stay overnight in a private room with their child. Where a baby has been stillborn or was an early fetal loss, careful thought needs to be given as to where the family might stay. While the mother might be eligible for midwifery care, it is clearly not appropriate for her to be in the same room as women who are either still pregnant or who have a live baby beside them.

OFFERING CHOICES

We have emphasised throughout this book that offering choices may enable bereaved people, whether an adult or child, to feel more in control of a devastating situation. Offering choices is not a 'once-only option'; families can take time to decide what they want over the following few days. As parents described in Chapter 3, these activities can represent continuing parental and family care for the child, reaffirm the finality of death and create memories for the future.

Some activities may not be immediately available, or even possible, for some families. Parents whose baby miscarries at 16 weeks of gestation may have very limited choices for touching or dressing their child because of the fragility of the baby's skin and lack of suitably sized clothing. Where a child has extensive injuries from a vehicle crash, the body may not be intact nor complete. Lord (1996) recommended that family members need to know exactly what the body will look like before going to see it. Sometimes, when the circumstances of death are unknown, there may be hospital policies about not leaving family members alone with the body of a child prior to postmortem or completion of police investigation. The assumption behind such policies is generally that information that might contribute to ascertaining the cause of death could be destroyed. In such circumstances, a nurse or midwife might clarify with senior management any particular requirements of the coroner, police or pathologist regarding family members having access to their child.

CARING FOR THEIR CHILD

The care that families may wish to show their dead child includes both physical and spiritual aspects. It is now common practice to offer the following choices to parents in maternity units:

- staying with their baby as long as they want
- washing and dressing their baby
- accompanying their baby to the mortuary
- bringing relatives (including children) to see the dead baby
- hand/foot prints, photographs, lock of hair
- taking their baby home.

Dent et al (1996) found that parents of older children who died in hospital wanted such choices but were not always offered them. Most were able to stay with their child, but only a quarter had been offered the chance to wash their child. The same number would have valued the opportunity. Half the parents had dressed the dead child but the majority of others would have chosen to do this if offered. Where possible, such choices are relevant to the entire family, including bereaved siblings who may appreciate the chance to see and touch their brother or sister.

SEEING THEIR CHILD

Families need to know what to expect if they choose to see their child at the time of death and subsequently. At the time of a sudden death, there may be changes to appearance resulting from injuries. In the case of a baby born with anencephaly or macerated skin having died in utero prior to birth, then the appearance may not match expected images of newborn babies. With this in mind, should all parents be encouraged to see and/or hold their child? As we noted in Chapter 6, information from two studies of mothers whose baby was stillborn suggests that such activities do not necessarily improve grieving outcomes for all women. As we have noted throughout the book, any form of care cannot be assumed to suit **all** parents or family members. Therefore, nurses and midwives need to consider ways to support family members to make decisions about what feels best for each individual. Most importantly, the shock of the sudden death does not mean that the decision to see the child is a 'once-only' choice. Family members can go home and then decide to return hours or days later to see their child. Children in the family may appreciate choices too. Clearly such choices will be shaped by the parents' beliefs. The information in Chapter 4 indicates that some siblings found it helpful to see the dead child after careful and gentle preparation. No child should be forced to view their sibling. If they choose to do so, it can be an opportunity for them to say goodbye and may reinforce the fact of death, both of which may help to make some sense of the death. Family members also need information over the following days, to appreciate that the appearance of their child will change. The skin often becomes 'woody' and firm to touch; if the body is stored in a mortuary, then it will feel cold.

If family members choose to see their child, nurses and midwives need to think how this will be organised (Speraw 1994). It requires setting the scene of the environment, surroundings, clothing and appearance:

- **environment**: a private and comfortable room, preferably with chairs, a carpet, possibly flowers and low lighting options
- **unnecessary equipment**: items such as intravenous cannulae should be removed unless these are required to be left in place for the postmortem
- **dressing the child**: for example using clothes provided by the family or of the correct size if born prematurely, or wrappings such as a silk handkerchief used to 'nest' and cover a very small fetus
- **appearance**: consider the possibility of covering up, where possible, injury or altered physical appearance such as anencephaly to allow families to explore and uncover it as they wish
- **surroundings of the child**: ensuring that the cot, bed or Moses basket is of an appropriate size to the child so that they are not 'lost' in it.

For many parents and family members who may never have seen a dead body before, it can be a fearful experience. An accompanying nurse or midwife can help them to focus on their child and not the fear. To help parents through these moments, health professionals can talk to the child, comment on how the child looks and ask the parents if they would like to touch the child.

When a child remains in hospital prior to a postmortem or is transferred to a funeral director's premises, families need to have the opportunity to visit their child. They will require details of whom to contact and where to visit. Where possible the same member of hospital staff should prepare the child for visiting by 'setting the scene' when the child is brought from the mortuary, welcoming the family and being available to stay with them while visiting. This can provide continuity of support. Such care may require a commitment from both individual health professionals and the health organisation to ensure that resources exist to support families to see their child.

TOKENS OF REMEMBRANCE

Previous chapters have discussed the importance placed by many families on having tokens of remembrance of the dead child. Dent et al (1996) found that hand and foot prints of older children who died were rarely offered to parents, a lock of hair was offered to only a quarter of parents and less than half the parents had been offered a photograph. Yet, on reflection, more than half the parents would have liked these tokens. Other comments from parents demonstrate the need for imagination and thoughtfulness.

> *I would have liked the nightie she died in. I was given one we took her to hospital in. I went home and washed some blood off it.*

> *We decided to leave a ring on her finger, but now we wish we had kept it for my wife to wear on a necklace. This suggestion would have been nice at the time as it is difficult to think straight.*

Preparation and consent

Taking photographs, locks of hair or nail clippings from a dead child, may not be acceptable to some people for personal or religious reasons. Before creating any tokens of remembrance, it is always important to talk with parents and receive their consent. Parents who indicate that they do not want photographs or other tokens of remembrance can be asked whether they would like such items collected and stored in the child's records. These can be available to the family on request at a later date. The discussion and decision needs to be fully documented.

To smooth the process of creating tokens of remembrance, it is useful to have the necessary resources available. White and Rosen (2000) described a resource that could be adapted to suit different practice settings. They developed a ready-prepared quilted memory box containing newborn outfit and hat, plastic bag for lock of hair, card and kit for hand/foot prints, booklets on grieving and information on support groups.

Photographs

As the earlier chapters indicated, photographs are often an important source of memories and conversations about the dead child. Many families want photographs of their child; some may be uncertain about having a photograph of a dead person and a few will decline for a range of reasons. Nurses and midwives have an important role both in offering and in assisting families to secure photographs that may have a lifelong value. This role includes choice of camera, number of photographs, the photographer and the picture composition. This is discussed in detail in Appendix 9.

Hand, foot and kiss prints

Hand and foot prints can generally be taken from any child and most babies who are of a gestational age, when a hand or foot has formed and is present. Where possible a 'pair' of hand or foot prints should be recorded. Some hospitals use inkless baby wipes with sensitised labels for imprints. It is possible to use inkpads to create the print but these, despite carefully cleaning with an alcohol wipe, may leave traces of ink. Parents need to be aware of this in advance. Other options include water-based paints, which may be easier to remove than ink. Kiss prints can be taken from a child's lips using lipstick. Hand and foot prints can be scanned into a computer and may be used as part of memory cards or on the order of service handed out at the funeral. Various 'cards' exist to make a special presentation format for the prints. Mutual help groups, hospitals and individual midwives produce such cards.

Locks of hair, nail clippings

Family members might like to obtain these themselves. For premature babies it may only be possible to secure a small amount of downy hair by using a dry-shave razor. It is useful to consider taking hair from the back of the head so that subsequent facial photographs will not show a gap in the hair.

Clothes

Many families want to keep a set of clothes worn by the child at death. Some may want to keep these unwashed clothes because the smell of the child may be an important memory for them. Some parents may wish to dress their child in clothes brought from home.

Personal records

Most parents do not ask for these on the day the child died but may seek them in the following weeks or months. Items requested may include: copies of case notes and records; radiographs (often taken as part of a postmortem), hospital identity bracelets, scan pictures of babies in utero, antenatal and labour cardiotocograph traces, and the postmortem report. Records are potential tokens of remembrance and, in rare instances, part of review inquiries into the circumstances of death. The fact that records are potential tokens of remembrance is a reminder of the need for documentation to be legible and to have sufficient detail to describe the care provided.

SPIRITUAL CARE

Many families have personal or religious beliefs that guide the activities and rituals that they wish to undertake with their child. These include staying with the child until the time of the funeral, having a blessing spoken by a spiritual leader, playing particular music or anointing the child with specific substances. Assumptions cannot be made that a family from a particular ethnic, religious or social group will always have certain beliefs and practices; there may be considerable diversity within groups. Where necessary, nurses and midwives can work with interpreters and community leaders to ask family members if there are activities that they wish to undertake. A current list of local clergy and other spiritual advisors needs to be available to assist health professionals respond to requests from the family for spiritual support. Most hospitals, and many individual health professionals, have established valuable links with local community and spiritual leaders who can offer such support to families. Where particular family requirements for the spiritual care of the child may conflict with legislative requirements, such as a post-mortem, then a medical practitioner and other relevant professionals may need to be involved to explore final options and decisions.

THE GIFT OF ORGAN OR TISSUE DONATION FOR TRANSPLANT

As the Paediatric Intensive Care Society (2002, p. 39) *Standards of bereavement care* indicate, most parents appreciate being told about any opportunity to donate the organs and tissues of their child for transplantation. Otherwise, they may wonder why they were not asked and even feel resentful at not having the choice (Dent et al 1996). Thomas (1999) described how important it was for parents whose baby was stillborn to have the choice of donating heart valves. In such situations, some parents may consider the organ as a 'gift' to another child. In all cases where organ donation is chosen, there must be a defined cause of death. When a child is diagnosed as brainstem dead and has a beating heart, then all major organs can be used provided there has been no previous history of infection or life-threatening disease. The following is a summary from discussions with a Transplant Coordinator (Bristol Hospitals, personal communication, 2003). Corneas and heart valves must be retrieved in the first 24 hours after death. Organs of babies under 6 months are not used because of lack of development. Tissues may be donated from babies of 37 weeks of gestation onwards and may include heart valves and corneas. Where there is any doubt about donation, the coroner or the local transplant coordinator should be contacted. Further information is available in the *Code of practice for the diagnosis of brain-stem death* (Department of Health 1998). The subject of donation needs to be broached by someone who is able to answer parents' questions and ensure that necessary processes for consent are undertaken. Like any major decision, parents may need time to see beyond their immediate personal grief to consider the wider issue of helping others.

TAKING THEIR CHILD HOME AFTER DEATH

Dent et al (1996) found that a small number of parents whose older children had died had been offered the choice of taking the body home. Many more parents wished that they had been given this choice. Provided the death has been confirmed, a postmortem is not required and/or the death certificate has been issued, parents may be able to take their child home if they desire. Transport may be either by an undertaker or parents may choose to make their own arrangements. In many maternity units in the UK, a casket is offered to the parents. When this is not available, a baby may be wrapped in a blanket and carried by a parent. An older, bigger child may pose greater problems for transportation, in which case, funeral directors may be more appropriate. If a car is used, a letter should be given to the driver in the event of being stopped or being involved in an accident. Some funeral directors recommend that a body is embalmed before going home. This process preserves body tissues and may have some value if the child is at home for several days, particularly in warmer weather when body tissues deteriorate. Otherwise, parents could consider placing the body of their child in a cool room without 24 hour central heating. Alternatively, some parents choose to visit their child at a funeral parlour until the day before the funeral, when the child is brought home and leaves for the funeral from home.

INVOLVEMENT OF THE CORONER AND POSTMORTEMS

The details in this section pertain to England and Wales and are determined by the Coroners Act (1988) and Birth and Deaths Registration Act (1953); both are available from www.hmso.gov.uk/acts. There is some variation in the registration processes in Scotland and Northern Ireland (see Registering the death, below). The following is a brief summary of the role of the coroner in relation to registration of deaths as described on the government website www.statistics.gov.uk/registration.

In some situations, deaths must be notified to the coroner before the death can be registered. These include when the cause of death is:

- unknown
- believed to be unnatural or suspicious
- a medical practitioner is unable to issue a medical certificate of the cause of death
- the deceased has not been seen by the medical practitioner issuing the certificate of cause of death nor has been seen in the 14 days prior to death
- death occurred during an operation.

In such cases, the medical practitioner will inform the coroner. The coroner is responsible for deciding if any further investigation is necessary. Until this time, the death cannot be registered by the registrar. The coroner's decisions may include:

- no further investigation necessary
- investigation of death circumstances
- postmortem by pathologist, preferably with a paediatric focus in cases of child death
- proceed to an inquest.

A coroner's officer, or police officer acting on the coroner's behalf, is likely to investigate the circumstances of death. This may involve an interview with the parents/other relevant witnesses and observation of the place of death. When babies have died for no obvious cause, investigation may include the removal of items of bedding for further examination. If the coroner decides no further action is needed, and a cause of death is certified, then the death can be registered (see p. 150). If the cause of death is confirmed by postmortem with no inquest, then the coroner confirms the cause of death and issues Pink Form B, which enables the death to be registered. If the case proceeds to inquest, then the coroner issues the death certificate and any certificates necessary for burial or cremation.

THE POSTMORTEM

In situations where a coroner requests a postmortem, families are not legally required to consent to the process (Coroner's Office Bristol, personal communication, 2003). However, families need to be prepared by an experienced health professional who is able to explain the situation and answer questions. In many localities, a paediatrician undertakes this role. For families whose personal beliefs mean that a postmortem is unacceptable or needs to be completed within a certain time period, then the relevant medical practitioner and coroner's officer need to meet with families to reach a solution. Following concerns raised about organ retention, during inquiries into practices at Alder Hey and Bristol hospitals, it may be possible for a partial postmortem to be carried out (Retained Organs Commission 2002). This is a detailed examination limited to a particular part of the body. Further information is available in *Human bodies: human choices* (Department of Health 2002).

Postmortems, or a range of investigations, may also be offered to families in circumstances where a coroner is not involved and the death is certified by the health professional at the birth. For example, investigations may offer information about the cause of stillbirth or early fetal death that may be preventable in a future pregnancy. Such investigations may not require a full postmortem and may include examination of specific organs or tissues including the placenta and analysis of infant/maternal blood. Time may be required to prepare organs for examination in which case the funeral may have to be delayed. This can be a cause of distress for families, who need to be advised of this possibility. Before signing a consent form for a full or partial postmortem, parents should be offered the opportunity to ask questions. They will also need to know when the results will be available and have an appointment to discuss these with a relevant practitioner such as a paediatrician or pathologist.

Information for parents about postmortems

Many people believe that postmortems are invasive and mutilating operations. Their perception is often based on watching television documentaries and medical dramas. In addition, recent media coverage since 1999 of organ retention without parental consent at hospitals in the UK has created further fears about postmortems.

This has become a concern for many parents, as Rose described in her story in Chapter 3. To help families to appreciate what a postmortem involves, the following information may be important. It will need to be adapted to suit local practices and circumstances of death. Further details are supplied in the Paediatric Intensive Care Society document *Standards for bereavement care* (2002, p. 24).

Why are postmortems necessary?   Postmortems are a legal requirement of any sudden death where the cause is not apparent. This applies to all people of any age and, therefore, is not targeted at the family personally. Postmortems are also available in other situations such as stillbirth.

What can postmortems offer?   Postmortems can provide valuable information about causes of death. In some situations, this may help to prevent the death of another child in the family or in a future pregnancy.

What is involved?   A pathologist, who is also a medical practitioner, undertakes postmortems carefully and respectfully. It generally involves two incisions: the length of the breastbone and at the back of the head. This allows the pathologist to examine body organs and tissues. On completion, the incisions are generally sutured and covered with an adhesive dressing. In the case of a small fetus it may not be possible to repair the incisions. The child will generally look as they did prior to the postmortem and it is possible for family members to see and hold their child after the postmortem.

When will it be done and the findings known?   Families need to know planned dates for postmortem and at what point the body might be released in order to plan for the funeral. Dent et al (1996) found that the majority of parents reported that the postmortem had been carried out on the day after death. A small number had to wait for up to 6 days for the results. This can be a difficult and testing time for the parents and family.

GIVING INFORMATION TO FAMILIES

In earlier chapters, we have discussed the personal and social resources that individuals use to make sense of what has happened when a child dies suddenly. Nurses and midwives are one social resource for families, providing both information and the opportunity to talk. The suddenness of the death can mean that everything is unfamiliar, unknown and bewildering for families. As Catherine described in Chapter 5, the world turns upside down. Parents may feel that they no longer have rights or choices over their child. Therefore, it is important that parents know the following information before they leave the hospital or before a child is taken from the place where they died.

Specific details may vary in different localities. It is important for nurses and midwives to know current details and arrangements to give to parents.

Where the child is.   Generally, a child is moved from the place where death was confirmed. If awaiting a postmortem, this may be to the hospital mortuary or another location. If the cause of death can be certified, the child may be transferred to a funeral parlour or go home with the parents.

What will happen to the child.   For example, will there be a postmortem and involvement of police or coroners' officers?

Where and when can parents see the child.   If the child is not going home with the parents, many hospitals and funeral directors provide 24-hour access to see a dead person, providing a time is arranged. This requires knowing **who** to contact to be able to arrange access.

Finally, it is important to indicate **who** will contact the parents about the death once they are at home. This varies according to local services and cause of death. It might include:

- a visit from the midwife the next day to offer both postnatal care to a newly delivered mother and bereavement follow-up for the parents
- a visit fom the health visitor (or equivalent) and/or GP, who will be informed of the death as soon as possible
- contact from a bereavement coordinator or social worker
- an appointment to see a paediatrician or obstetrician to discuss postmortem findings.

This ongoing contact from health professionals offers family members one form of social support to cope with the sudden death of their child.

INFORMATION ON PRACTICAL ISSUES

Family members may lack knowledge of grieving (Dent et al 1996). For many people, this may be their first experience of the death of someone close to them. The consistent message from families, mutual help groups and research is that parents want information to enable them to understand what is happening. We recommend that an information pack is given to all parents before they leave the hospital. Written information can be helpful for family members, who may remember only limited amounts of information as they try and assimilate the news of their child's sudden death. The pack could include the following information:

- location and access to their dead child if they remain in the hospital mortuary, and details of whom to contact to be able to visit the child
- registering the death (and birth if necessary)
- postmortems (if appropriate)
- choices for arranging a funeral
- contact details and support available from local bereavement agencies and mutual help groups (see following section)
- details of books of remembrance and regular memorial services that may be offered in the local hospital or community
- a follow-up appointment to see any relevant professionals, such as obstetrician/ paediatrician, to discuss the circumstances of death and/or postmortem findings (in some situations parents may wish to discuss the relevance of such information

for a future pregnancy); where possible parents should be offered the choice of a home or hospital visit

- grief and how it may affect family members differently (see following section).

It is useful to give parents at least **two** copies of the information; a copy for parents to keep and a spare copy for other family members or friends. The value of such a resource is that it can be revisited time and again. Much of this information is available in leaflets from bereavement agencies and mutual help groups (Appendices 1 and 2). In addition, a short letter could be included giving information relevant to the local area. In some areas, there may be a need to work with communities to produce information to suit the needs of particular ethnic groups in the locality.

INFORMATION ABOUT GRIEF

While, 'need-to-know' information at the time of the child's death may be limited, supporting written information can be more extensive and include material on helping grieving family members over time. Key information, which nurses and midwives could offer, includes:

- the **range** of 'common' feelings and reactions to bereavement, which can be extensive and frightening
- the **physical** aspect of grief, such as inability to sleep or eat, which is often overlooked
- the **diversity** of responses to the child's death, which may mean that family members feel and behave very differently to each other; this includes information on grieving children.

INFORMATION ABOUT MUTUAL HELP GROUPS AND BEREAVEMENT AGENCIES

As we discussed in Chapters 2 and 6, various forms of social support exist for bereaved family members. To enable members to access these resources, they need information about support that is available in the form of information, 24-hour phone lines, befrienders and groups. While some will not choose to access these, others may do so sooner or later. Some people may want to meet with a befriender but find it too hard to make a telephone call to an unknown person. Family or friends might do this on their behalf. Contact details of various national organisations for parents and siblings are included in Appendices 1 and 2. Some of the resources available for siblings, parents and grandparents are listed in Appendices 3–6. It is worth finding out about local resources so that contact details can be included in any information given to families.

COMMUNICATION AND LIAISON WITH OTHER PROFESSIONALS AND AGENCIES

Midwives and nurses work alongside many other professionals who are involved in the lives of families. Practitioners, such as neonatalogists, paediatricians, GPs, health visitors and social workers need to know about the child's death. They may be part of ongoing follow-up with the bereaved family and offer another resource for grieving family members. The health professionals involved around the time of death have an important role to notify other agencies and health professionals about the death. Nurses and midwives need to be aware of any constraints regarding sharing information about family members. In general, families appreciate knowing that other agencies and health professionals will be contacted on their behalf. This can alert other health professionals currently involved with the family to contact the family. It may also avoid further distress for the family, who might otherwise be contacted unwittingly by someone who does not know the child is dead. It is also important to have a process to contact local or national child health databases, which issue automatic reminders for screening visits. In some localities, there may need to be processes to advise research projects in which the child was participating. Otherwise, as Rose described in Chapter 3, families may experience unnecessary distress. To assist parents to cope with the shock of the news, nurses and midwives might consider asking parents whether they would like anyone informed of the death. This might include their workplace and could enable colleagues and employers to offer acknowledgement and support to the parents.

REGISTERING THE DEATH

The following summary details are relevant to England Wales and offer a brief summary. Further information is available from the government website www.statistics.gov.uk/registration, which provides links to information about registration processes in Scotland and Northern Ireland. Clearly, the amount of information bereaved parents can cope with at the time of death is limited. Some will want to know extensive details. Others will need further information in the following days. All families may appreciate being given written information and this is often part of the booklets provided by mutual help groups (Appendix 1).

After any death, it is necessary for a cause of death to be confirmed and for the death to be registered. In many situations, a medical practitioner issues a medical certificate of cause of death. This is given to a family member, who will then register the death. The certificate must be filled in correctly and accurately to avoid any delay in registering the death, with the name of the doctor written in capitals to enable the registrar to identify the doctor concerned. In the case of a stillborn baby, a midwife may complete the forms necessary to confirm birth and death. A stillbirth needs to be registered within 3 months of birth. In other situations, once a cause of death has been confirmed, families need to register the death within 5 days at the office of the Registrar of Births, Deaths and Marriages. The contact details are in the local phone directory. While deaths are registered in the district where they occurred, it is possible to take the information to the registrar in another district who will then send it to the registrar of the district of death. In the case of a baby, both the birth and death can be registered at the same time. If the parents are not married, then both will need to attend if they wish the father's name to be on the birth and death certificates. Relatives or someone present at the death can register a death. As it is important that the registrar enters details correctly, it may be appropriate for some families whose first language is not English to take an interpreter to assist them check the information. Once the death is registered the registrar issues:

- a death certificate (currently £3.50)
- a certificate for cremation or burial, which is a requirement for these to proceed
- BD8 for Department of Social Security to cancel child benefit.

Certificates of birth and death can be important tokens of remembrance; many parents place these in a memory box or book. The gestational age at which the death of a stillborn baby can be registered varies in different countries; it is 24 weeks in England and Wales. For babies who do not receive a certificate, many midwives offer families a card confirming details of birth and death. Commemorative cards are also provided by mutual help groups.

THE FUNERAL: CREMATION OR BURIAL

As some parents described in Chapter 3, hearing the news of a child's sudden death may mean that it is difficult to think, ask questions or plan for anything. Other parents will want to know what is going to happen and start planning the funeral. To accommodate the needs of different parents, it is advisable that nurses and midwives discuss these options with those who are interested and ensure that everyone has written information that can be accessed in the following days. Various agencies provide information leaflets about funerals (Appendix 1). Some options for the service are listed in Appendix 10.

As the stories of Rose (Ch. 3) and Jenny (Ch. 5) illustrate, choices about burial, cremation and the funeral are a central part of grieving the death of a child. None of the choices are easy decisions, since all reinforce the fact that the child has died. A funeral director, family members and/or the hospital chaplain may help in arranging the funeral. Choosing a funeral director may be by personal recommendation of family/friends or from the local telephone directory. Health professionals can encourage the family to take time to consider the various choices and feel comfortable in what they decide. There is no requirement to rush to have a funeral within a couple of days of death. This is particularly important if the parents are uncertain about interment options. For example, when a baby who is a twin or multiple birth dies, and the parents do not know whether other sibling(s) may die. In some situations where the death is investigated, the funeral may be delayed until the coroner issues certificates of cremation or burial.

When families experience miscarriage, the situation is not as definitive as when a baby is born after 24 weeks of gestation with subsequent registration of birth and death, followed by burial or cremation. As Moulder (2001, p. 64) noted, for babies born prior to 24 weeks of gestation without signs of life, *The question of disposal, a horrible word but there really is no other, is a difficult and sensitive one.* If a woman has been admitted to hospital, disposal arrangements, generally involving inciner-ation, can be made by the hospital. The sensitivity of any arrangements varies according to different localities. It may include incineration separate from other hospital waste, a memorial service and scattering of ashes at a local cemetery. Nurses and midwives need to know what is available in their locality since parents generally want to know what will happen. Alternatively, the family can make arrangements themselves for the remains to be buried or cremated. Many families choose this option when the pregnancy ends as a late loss around 15–23 weeks of gestation. The family can approach a local funeral director, crematorium or cem-etery. Generally, families need a letter from a health professional stating that the pregnancy ended before 24 weeks with no signs of life at delivery. Some families who experience early miscarriage, less than 12 weeks of gestation, make choices to bury the remains under a plant in the garden. We have also met families who have chosen to place the remains in a plant pot, which can be taken with the family if they subsequently move house.

Many funeral directors offer their basic service free of cost to families whose child dies under the age of 16 years. This generally includes costs of organising the funeral and the coffin, but there is likely to be a charge for cars or extra services. When all services are charged, it may be advisable to get several quotes. Family and friends can assist with this. Funeral directors will take time to talk through various choices. However, it is possible for families to organise a funeral without the services of a funeral director. The hospital chaplain will be aware of local firms, or family and friends can make enquiries. Some of the choices that fami-lies might wish to consider include location, service, tokens of remembrance and interment.

FUNERAL OR MEMORIAL SERVICE

As we have noted earlier, some families will want to talk about options with health professionals soon after hearing the news of the sudden death. Others will want such information in the days following the death. Many parents, such as Rose, appreciate being offered ideas about the funeral so that they can make the 'best' choices possible for their child. Nurses and midwives are in a position to offer such information and share ideas that have been used by other families. Choices of loca-tion may include hospital chapel, local church, crematorium chapel and funeral directors' premises. Some families choose to have a memorial service in their own garden or at a place of special significance to them. Many parents involve grand-parents and other children in making family decisions about the form of the service. Choices that might be considered are included in Appendix 10. As the com-ments of family members indicated in earlier chapters, the funeral can be a source of tokens of remembrance of the child. These can include dried flowers, a tribute list of people who attended and a video or audiotape. Some parents send memory cards with a personalised photograph or image of their child. Details inside the card could include birth and death dates, commemorative verse or artwork.

CHOICES OF INTERMENT

In the case of babies born before the age of viability, many hospitals have arrangements for the respectful disposal of their bodies in a designated area, which parents can visit. Nurses and midwives need to be aware of the practices of the hospital in which they work. Some funeral directors will assist towards the cost of a baby's funeral; others will pay the full amount for a child up to 16 years. Otherwise, parents generally have to fund costs of burial or cremation themselves unless they are eligible for a social security grant (Form SF200 Funeral Payment from the Social Fund).

BURIAL

Burial can be in a cemetery or churchyard. Some churches have policies as to who can be buried and where they can be buried in a churchyard. This sometimes excludes babies who are stillborn or born before 24 weeks. Either the pastor of the churchyard or the local funeral director can advise on the regulations that apply. Burial in a cemetery may be in a designated area for children, the general area or in a family plot. Some parents may want to bury their child or the ashes on private ground. There are national regulations for such practices with which funeral directors are familiar. After burial, some families choose headstones, sculptures and plaques to mark the physical space surrounding their child. These may need to meet requirements of the churchyard or cemetery in terms of size or appearance. Costs for burial include any charges for the land with extra charges for digging the grave and upkeep of the area.

CREMATION

Crematoria may charge for their service but usually babies under 1 year are cremated free. Some crematoria state that there will be no ashes remaining from a baby. In this instance, parents should be informed so that they are prepared or they may wish to make alternative arrangements. Parents also need to consider where they would like either to scatter or to keep the ashes. Families can generally choose to place a plaque to the memory of their child on a memory wall at local cemeteries or in a designated Garden of Remembrance for children.

SUMMARY

Caring for families around the time of death can be a privilege. Nurses and midwives are involved in the lives of families at a time when their family world has been torn apart. The discussion of the care at this time lays foundations for ongoing follow-up discussed in Chapter 8. Bereavement care requires adequate organisational resources to enable professionals to offer confident, sensitive and imaginative care. These issues are discussed further in Chapter 9.

SUMMARY POINTS

- Parents and their families may remember the care given by hospital staff to them and their child for years to come. Thus nurses and midwives need to offer sensitive, and compassionate care at all times.
- This support **lays the foundations** for follow-up bereavement care (p. 134).
- Parents need to be offered choices and encouraged to take time to make decisions. This may help to give them a sense of control at a time when their world has turned upside down.
- Where possible, parents should be offered the chance to have tokens of remembrance of their child.
- If a postmortem is planned, parents need to have a full explanation and the opportunity to ask questions.
- Parents need both verbal and written information on a wide range of subjects, including registering the death, grief and sources of support in the local community, such as mutual help groups.
- Health professionals who provide care at the time of death need to inform other agencies and professionals to enable follow-up care for the family.

REFERENCES

Dent A, Condon L, Fleming P et al 1996 A study of bereavement care after sudden and unexpected death. Archives of Disease in Childhood 74: 522–526

Department of Health 1998 Code of practice: for diagnosis of brain-stem death. Department of Health, London

Department of Health 2002 Human bodies, human choices: the law on human organs and tissue in England and Wales. Department of Health, London

Gibran K 1980 The prophet. Heineman, London

Henrietta C, Vanbrunt PF 1982 Sudden paediatric death: meeting the needs of family and staff. Nurse Educator Winter: 13–16

Hindmarch C 2000 On the death of a child, 2nd edn. Radcliffe Medical Press, Oxford

Korth SK 1988 Behavioural issues: unexpected death in the emergency department – supporting the family. Journal of Emergency Nursing,14: 302–304

Lord JH 1996 America's number one killer: vehicular crashes. In: Doka K (ed) Living with grief after sudden loss. Taylor Francis, Philadelphia, PA, p 25–41

Moulder C 2001 Miscarriage: women's experiences and needs, 2nd edn. Routledge, London

Paediatric Intensive Care Society 2002 Standards for bereavement care. Available from Secretary, Dr C Stack. PICU, Sheffield Children's Hospital, Western Bank, Sheffield S10 2TH, UK

Retained Organs Commission National Health Service 2002 Annual Report April 2001–March. Retained Organs Commission National Health Service, PO Box 32794, London

Soreff S 1984 Sudden death in the emergency department: a comprehensive approach for families, emergency medical technicians and emergency department staff. Critical Care Medicine 10: 254–258

Speraw S 1994 The experience of miscarriage: how couples define quality in health care delivery. Journal of Perinatology 14: 208–215

Thomas J 1999 A baby's death – helping parents make difficult choices. The Practising Midwife 2: 16–19

Von Bloch L 1996 Breaking the bad news when sudden death occurs. Social Work in Health Care 23: 91–97

Warland J 2000 The midwife and the bereaved family. Ausmed, Ascot Vale, Australia

White D, Rosen J 2000 A memory box for baby Chandler. AORN Journal 72: 280–282

Wright B 1996 Sudden death, 2nd edn. Churchill livingstone, Edinburgh

USEFUL SOURCES FOR NURSES AND MIDWIVES

Hindmarch C 2000 On the death of a child, 2nd edn. Radcliffe Medical Press, Oxford

Kohner N, Henley A 2001 When a baby dies, 2nd edn. Routledge, London

Mander R 1994 Loss and bereavement in childbearing. Blackwell, Oxford

Moulder C 2001 Miscarriage: women's experiences and needs, 2nd edn. Routledge, London

Warland J 2000 The midwife and the bereaved family. Ausmed, Ascot Vale, Australia

Wright B 1996 Sudden death, 2nd edn. Churchill Livingstone, London.

Supporting bereaved families over time

> *There are always two parties to a death; the person who dies and the survivors who are bereaved ... and in the apportionment of suffering, the survivor takes the brunt.*
>
> Arnold Toynbee
> *Cited by Stillion 1996*

INTRODUCTION

In Chapter 7, we considered the role of nurses and midwives, often working in a hospital setting, who provide initial support and care for bereaved family members at the time of a child's sudden death. The way family members are supported from the outset may have long-lasting effects. Toynbee described one perspective of family members' pain and distress in the opening quotation. Many family members describe their feelings worsening in the first 6 months, by which time there may be little support from family and friends. In addition, as parents described in Chapter 3, follow-up from health professionals is often absent or variable (Finlay & Dallimore 1991, Dent et al 1996). Part of the responsibilities of nurses and midwives involved at the time of death is to inform other health professionals who can continue to give support to the grieving family in the following months. Chapter 6 outlined general considerations for professional practice when working with bereaved family members. This chapter explores considerations for practice in the weeks and months after the death. The content is informed by material predominantly focused on sudden child death, which was discussed in earlier chapters, including family members' comments, research and our clinical experience. In order to keep the focus on practical considerations, we have only included references to key materials. As we have discussed in earlier chapters, these considerations cannot be generalised to **all** bereaved families who experience the sudden, unexpected death of a child; the ideas need to be adapted to suit the diversity of situations and individuals. Adaptation requires professional judgement, flexibility and imagination. It also requires nurses and midwives to use knowledge of research relevant to the particular group of people with whom they are working.

THE CONTEXT AND PURPOSE OF BEREAVEMENT CARE

CONTEXT OF CARE

Rando (1986a,b, 1996) has indicated that grieving may be different or complicated in some circumstances of bereavement, such as sudden death or death of a child. For families whose child dies suddenly, these two situations are combined. Riches and Dawson (2000, p. 132) noted that some deaths are '*difficult*' to adjust to and there may be limited resources available to family members for a range of social and cultural reasons. For example, the stigma associated with violent death (Redmond 1996) and the lack of social value placed on a miscarriage or death of a baby (Malacrida 1998, Moulder 2001) may mean that there is little acknowledgement or support for the family. This was illustrated in some of the comments from parents and grandparents in Chapters 3 and 5.

So, should all families whose child dies suddenly receive follow-up care? Some families will feel that they have sufficient resources to cope. Others, as Dent et al (1996) identified, appreciate ongoing support from health professionals. Therefore, we believe that all families who experience the sudden death of a child should be offered the opportunity to have follow-up care. We appreciate that some health professionals may already be severely taxed with existing workloads. As we noted in Chapter 6, provision of bereavement care may require review of existing funding and resources in health provider organisations.

The provision of health care within a defined geographical area or within particular funding targets may preclude offering home visiting to all family members such as grandparents and others. As Jane described in Chapter 5, care is often focused on the parents; therefore, we have tended to use 'parents' in this chapter while recognising that such care can apply to other family members.

It is also likely that many bereaved parents, whose child dies in particular circumstances, may not receive follow-up care. For example, Moulder (2001) noted that many do not receive follow-up care after miscarriage. Nurses and midwives might consider whether there is follow-up for all bereaved families in their area. What happens to parents after an early miscarriage if they are not part of the caseload of a midwife or health visitor? What happens when a young baby dies? Does the midwife offer follow-up care or is there a handover to the health visitor? Who cares for families after the death of an older child where there are no younger siblings? Having considered some of the tensions about the extent and context of follow-up, nurses and midwives need to consider their goal, role and scope of practice (see Chapter 6).

PURPOSE OF CARE

In earlier chapters we proposed that nurses, midwives and health visitors are one of the social resources available to bereaved individuals and can assist them to cope with, and make some sense of, the death. Follow-up care demonstrates to a bereaved family the concern and compassion of other human beings. This may be extremely important to parents and other family members, especially if they receive little acknowledgement and support from friends and colleagues. We suggested that a companion role (Murray 1993) may be appropriate for some health professionals, and that a broad goal for practice is the promotion of the health and well-being of individuals and their family.

The considerations proposed in this chapter need to be located within a framework for practice (p. 117) with an appreciation of theoretical perspectives of grief. In Chapter 6, we noted that the ideas discussed in Chapter 2 can provide nurses and midwives with an appreciation of the complexity of grief. Riches and Dawson (2000) proposed that these perspectives offer maps of grieving, although, as we described on page 115, the maps cannot be used prescriptively to determine how all people will grieve. Rather, they offer a way to understand that different people go on different journeys as they cope with the meaning that the death has for their lives. Some nurses and midwives find useful maps to assist with follow-up including Worden's (1991) tasks of grieving (see p. 28), Rando's (1993) 6 'R' processes (p. 30) and the work of Riches and Dawson (2000) and Stroebe and Schut (2001).

The language that nurses and midwives use to describe grief needs to be considered carefully. Words such as 'adjust', 'adapt', 'accept', 'get over' have differing meanings to grieving people and some may be unacceptable. For example, one mother was adamant that she did not ever want to *accept* the death of her child because it meant for her that she had *agreed with* or *acquiesced to* the event.

Working with others: who is the key person?

Sometimes several agencies, including health professionals, are involved with a bereaved family. This may have benefits for the family but it can also lead to fragmentation of care and confusion, as some bereaved mothers described in the study of de Montigny, Beaudet and Dumas (1996). In such cases, it may be helpful to have a key worker who liaises with relevant professionals and who holds the primary responsibility for follow-up care of the family. Parents may want to choose their key worker. In the UK, depending on the age at death and other family circumstances, the midwife or health visitor could be suited to this role. An existing relationship may offer foreknowledge of the family and a familiar face for the parents. Both professionals have a focus on the physical and mental well-being of family members and have access to other professionals where necessary. Where multiple professionals are involved with a family, it may be useful to obtain the parents' consent for information about the family to be shared between different agencies to assist in planning care, such as who is visiting the family and when. With families whose first language is not English, the key worker's role may also include liaison with interpreters and relevant community leaders.

INFORMING THE WIDER COMMUNITY

Many nurses and midwives have involvement with a range of community groups from play centres to schools. The sudden death of a child creates a ripple of bereavement that extends beyond families to such groups. These may include other parents, teachers and friends of the child. Health professionals might assist staff in community groups to inform other children and families about the death. Where possible, this needs to be done in consultation with the bereaved family so that information is clear, accurate and acceptable to them. Hindmarch (2000) provided valuable examples of 'scripts' that can be read and then discussed with the target audience. Key information could include:

- what has happened
- when it happened
- acknowledgement of the distress felt by family and audience caused by the death
- funeral details, requests from the family (e.g. to visit at home before the funeral).

Discussion might also identify planned activities of the group to mark the death. These may vary from classmates and teachers attending the funeral to sending flowers on behalf of the group. Some schools and play centres create memorials to the child, such as planting a tree; others create memory books of their experiences with the child and give these to the parents. Health professionals can affirm the death and suggest ways to say goodbye to the child. The extent of ongoing professional support for children at community groups varies according to availability of services and cause of death. It may include 'post-vention' programmes for schools after youth suicide (Stillion 1996) or specialist trauma counsellors attending a school following a disaster.

PLANNED CARE: HOME VISITING AND BEREAVEMENT ASSESSMENT

HOME VISITING

Home visiting offers families the advantage of meeting in their own familiar sur-roundings and not in the potentially strange and stressful environment of hospitals or health centres. Recent small studies in the USA and the UK indicate that bereaved parents who wanted home follow-up found such visits valuable (Gaines et al 1996, Dent 2002). The extent of home visiting will vary according to the needs of the family. For example, Dent (2002) found that health visitors visited on average five times over the first 3 month period since the death, spending around 4 hours on average over that time with families. Between visits, health visitors contacted parents by phone and/or saw them in surgeries. Home visiting combined with other ways of keeping in contact with family members offers flexibility for everyone and may also mean that follow-up can be offered within existing funding resources.

Contract of care

The timing of the first visit will depend on the family and might be at the end of the first week after the death. It is valuable to make contact prior to the visit to acknowledge the death and to arrange a time for visiting. During the first visit, the purpose of follow-up care needs to be explained to ensure that the parent(s) under-stand the health professional's role. Otherwise some parents may be uncertain about the reason for the visit(s). In effect this explanation forms a contract of care and might include indicating:

- the purpose of visits (e.g. assessment, listening, offering information, ideas for coping)
- approximate length of visits (e.g. 1 hour in length)
- expected frequency of visits
- that bereavement follow-up is finite and does end
- contact details for the health professional.

Some parents may decline any follow-up contact or may repeatedly not be available at an agreed time. If this is the case, telephoning or leaving a note may be appropri-ate. Any attempts to contact the family need to be documented. Some families may not want visits and will choose other resources to assist their bereavement. In this instance, their decision should be respected while ensuring that the parents have been given relevant information about other support (see information pack details, p. 148). In some situations, various agencies are involved with the family for rea-sons other than bereavement follow-up, for example where there are concerns about the well-being of a family member. In such a case standard practices to ensure contact with the family will be followed. Sometimes parents move temporarily to be with relatives after the death. It is worth waiting several weeks before assuming that non-response to letters and phone calls means that they do not want a follow-up visit.

How long should a visit last?

The key to effective visiting is generally quality not quantity. We suggest that visits should, if at all possible, last no more than an hour. This is often long enough for the bereaved parent to cope with, and for the health professional to concentrate fully on what is being said by the bereaved parent. From the outset, the nurse or midwife could make it clear that the visit will last up to an hour and during that time they will concentrate on what is happening for the parent after the death. Making boundaries can be useful to both parties. Sometimes the bereaved parent may want to detain the professional either by words or tears. Depending on the situation, it may be appropriate to continue to end the visit and arrange a time for another visit. Maintaining the agreed ending time can help both the parent and health professional to focus on the purpose of follow-up during the agreed visiting time. When a parent has been left in tears, the nurse or midwife could phone later in the day to see how the parent is feeling and to reaffirm that health professionals are accessible.

What is involved in a visit?

The basis of any health professional's practice is to make an assessment of a situation using information gained from observation and, where possible, conversation with the client. This equally applies to working with bereaved families. When working with family members, we support the premise of Riches and Dawson (2000), outlined in Chapter 2, that individuals actively seek to make sense of what has happened to them and they use personal, social and cultural resources to do so. Therefore, assessment care can involve asking parents how they think they are coping and helping them to identify stressors and potential resources for their grief.

Therapists and psychiatrists have developed various assessment tools (e.g. Raphael 1984, pp. 363–367, Rando 1986c, pp. 354–364) to provide care suited to the bereaved individual. In the following section, we present an assessment tool used by UK health visitors. The UK health visitors who used it to plan care, and the parents who received the care, evaluated the tool favourably in a randomised controlled trial. A summary of this trial is presented on page xxvii and a fuller description is available in Dent (2002). Although only health visitors in the UK to-date have used the tool, other nurses and midwives could consider using, or adapting it, within their practice.

BEREAVEMENT ASSESSMENT

The bereavement assessment tool (Appendix 11) serves three main purposes for health professionals.

It provides a structure on which to base care and continuing contact.   This can help nurses and midwives feel confident about having a beginning point to their follow-up care, which may lessen the possibility of families feeling unsupported and isolated.

It stresses the uniqueness of each death.   It can help to reaffirm for health professionals the diversity of grief and the unique meanings that sudden child death can have for family members.

It helps to identify stressors.   These may be identified by bereaved parents, nurses and midwives and their acknowledgement can assist family members to use resources to reduce them, wherever possible. This can help bereaved family members to feel more in control, which may lessen the potential detrimental consequences of bereavement on physical and mental health.

The tool needs to be viewed for what it is, a tool that can assist practice. It can never replace professional judgement, interpretation of the information gained and skilled communication. Consequently, it is not a checklist; it is a beginning point for planning visits.

The tool is divided into sections that assist in identifying stresses within the family; these may be physical, psychological, sociocultural or spiritual. It was developed with reference to various writings (Worden 1983, Lazarus & Folkman 1984, Raphael 1984, Stroebe, Stroebe & Hanson 1993, Riches & Dawson 1996a,b) and is congruent with the idea of individuals using resources (Riches & Dawson, 2000). It is based on three assumptions, which have been discussed in previous chapters.

Integrated nature of grief.   The meaning a death holds for an individual is unique, encompassing all aspects of an individual's physical, mental, social and spiritual well-being. Bereaved people have a range of personal resources, such as beliefs and previous experiences, which can help them to cope with the changes that bereavement brings to their lives.

Individuals within a family.   Individuals do not grieve in isolation. This was apparent in the stories and comments of family members in the preceding chapters. Bereaved individuals are members of a family; this is the context within which the child dies. The death means that all family members are bereaved and the entire family world is changed in terms of roles, relationships and beliefs.

Social resources.   Support can help to decrease the effects of a stressful life event on psychological well-being. There are different forms of support such as emotional (listening and talking), practical (helping out) and informational (new ideas and ways of understanding the experience). Therefore, family, friends, health professionals, other carers, colleagues and acquaintances in local communities can all be viewed as resources for the bereaved individual.

Use of the tool

Before visiting families, the tool can be used as a framework to remind health professionals of the importance of awareness of the family and the stresses that might be present. We would suggest that the assessment tool (Appendix 11) is not used as a series of questions during the first visit. It could be somewhat daunting for parents to be presented with a whole range of questions soon after the shock of the death. At the first visit, it can be useful to listen to whatever is important to family members. Listening, being with and inviting people to tell a story of what is happening to them are valuable strategies in practice. They can offer acknowledgement of loss and concern for the bereaved person. It is also likely that listening to parents provides answers of relevance to the assessment tool.

The tool can help nurses and midwives to appreciate the diversity of responses, but it can only reflect the perception of the person answering the questions. This is usually the parents, or the mother alone. Consequently, the tool does not provide the detail of information that would be required to work with all family members as a family therapist might. However, there is value in using the tool with individual family members, who may find it helps them to appreciate that other family members view the bereavement in different ways. Some parents have appreciated reading through the tool as a means to help them to think about how they and their family are coping. To accompany the tool, a pictorial representation of the family can be used, which might be in the form of a genogram (e.g Lindsey & Elsegood 1996, pp. 131–134). This can help to identify the range of family members and sources of support both within and outside the family. Asking parents and children how they see their family and the people who help them can be part of the initial follow-up visit. Both health professionals and family members may gain insights into available resources and the relationships within the family.

How does the assessment tool assist in planning care?

Follow-up care can be planned using two sources of assessment. First, the family member's self assessment; some aspects of the tool may have guided them to have new insights about how they are coping. Second, the health professional's assessment based on the information gathered by using the tool as a framework to listen and ask questions. As in any situation in clinical practice, assessment involves interpreting information with recognition of the surrounding context. The latter includes the family structure, time since death and changes in the family member's responses or stressors. This is then integrated with knowledge from research, theory and practice. Conclusions might be recorded using the structured care plan at the end of the tool (Appendix 11) or as narrative written documentation. Identification of stressors, issues and resources form the basis of planning care. Care in this context, we believe, is about assisting people to cope with the death using a range of personal and social resources. Therefore, the nurse or midwife might make suggestions about coping strategies, provide information or arrange a meeting for the parents to discuss their unanswered questions with relevant professionals. These considerations for practice are discussed further, in this chapter and in Chapter 6. Some are illustrated in the following case study (Box 8.1), which describes how the tool may assist family members and the health professional to identify, prioritise and respond to stressors. There is an accompanying pictorial representation of the family, drawn by the health professional (Fig. 8.1). The case study does not represent any particular situation from practice; it is a fictionalised account of issues that we have encountered across a range of different situations.

Box 8.1   The use of the bereavement tool to identify, prioritise and respond to stressors

Three year old Gemma died unexpectedly in hospital from meningitis. When Susan, her health visitor, heard the news from the hospital, she telephoned Jane, Gemma's mother. Susan arranged to visit the family 2 days later, when Jane and her mother were at home.

First visit

Ben, Gemma's father, had gone to work for the afternoon. Nathan, Gemma's 8-year-old brother, had asked to go to school that day. Susan talked with Jane and her mother about what had been happening to the family, how they each felt and what they were concerned about. This enabled Susan to make an assessment of needs, guided by the assessment tool. Key information that she identified:

- Jane was crying incessantly, unable to eat or sleep and uncertain how to 'deal' with her partner's anger
- Jane's mother, who had travelled some distance from her own home, was becoming tired trying to carry on with household activities; she felt unable to console Jane
- Ben was feeling angry about Gemma's death, blaming the care offered at the hospital
- Nathan had been told about the death but did not want to talk about it with his parents; Jane and Ben were uncertain whether he should go to the funeral.

Susan talked with Jane and her mother about:

- recognising the physical effects of grief and the need to care for themselves; the range and intensity of feelings people have when they are grieving, including Ben's anger
- offering Nathan the choice of going to the funeral, preparing him for this and giving him an opportunity to talk about Gemma when he was ready.

Susan offered written information about the grief of parents, siblings and grandparents with accompanying contact details for a local mutual help group. She arranged for the family's GP to visit the next day. The GP prescribed some sleeping pills to help Jane to rest in the short term and discussed the circumstances of Gemma's death with Ben and Jane. Jane accepted Susan's offer to contact Nathan's teacher to ensure that the school felt able to support him. Before leaving, Susan arranged to visit a week after the funeral. She apologised for not being able to attend the funeral because of being out of town on work commitments. Susan encouraged Jane to contact her in the meantime with any further questions and concerns.

Second visit

Ben was again at work. Jane said she felt calmer and had taken sleeping tablets for only three nights to get to sleep. She felt she had coped well

Box 8.1
Continued

with the funeral. Her mother had gone home and had appreciated the information on grieving grandparents. Jane felt that the meeting with the GP had been helpful for herself and Ben, who now seemed less angry. Nathan had decided to go to the funeral and sometimes he did talk about Gemma. Jane's main concern was how to spend her days, which felt empty now that Gemma had gone.

Susan identified that Jane was coping with some everyday activities. She asked whether Jane had other people to talk to about Gemma. Jane said that she had good friends, but others avoided the subject. Susan asked Jane to tell her about Gemma. Jane talked for nearly an hour about her daughter's life and death, the good times and the difficult ones. They looked at photographs of the family together and talked about how Gemma would always be part of their family. Before leaving, Susan asked whether there was anything that Jane thought might assist the family at the moment. Jane said that she would like to talk to another bereaved mother but could not pluck up the courage to phone the local group. Susan offered to telephone on her behalf to ask if a befriender might visit. Susan arranged to visit again 2 weeks later.

Third visit

Jane said how much she had enjoyed talking to Susan about Gemma. She commented that talking with the befriender had helped to share some of the pain that no one else seemed to understand. She could talk about Gemma to her mother on the phone, but Ben would not talk about Gemma with herself or Nathan. She found this bewildering and frustrating. Susan identified that Jane and Ben were coping in different ways with Gemma's death. She discussed differences in the ways that people grieve and commented that many men cope mainly by keeping busy and women tend to cope by talking about the loss more. Susan suggested that Jane might mention this to Ben. It might also assist him to appreciate the differences in grieving. Susan asked if there were activities that Jane and Ben could do together, not necessarily to talk about Gemma but to share time in each other's company.

Overview of the following months

The visits continued over the following months. Stressors that Jane identified in her discussion with Susan included:

- how to keep Gemma's memory alive when friends did not want to talk about her
- what to do with Gemma's belongings
- how to cope with Nathan who was bullying other children at school
- what to do on the anniversary of Gemma's death.

Susan listened, offering suggestions and written information that might be of interest. She encouraged Jane to go to a local mutual help group,

Box 8.1
Continued

where Jane found a place to talk, to listen to others and gain new ways of making sense of her experience. On the anniversary of Gemma's death, Susan sent a card to Jane and Ben saying that she was thinking of them. A month later she met Jane, who felt that she no longer needed Susan to visit. Jane was now involved in the local mutual help group, was working in the family business for 3 days a week alongside Ben and sometimes was able to talk to Ben about Gemma. She thought that while she still had bad days and weeks, there were also times when she did not feel the pain as deeply all the time. She could think about things in the future. They agreed that Jane could always contact Susan if she had concerns or questions.

Figure 8.1
Pictorial representation of a family using a genogram

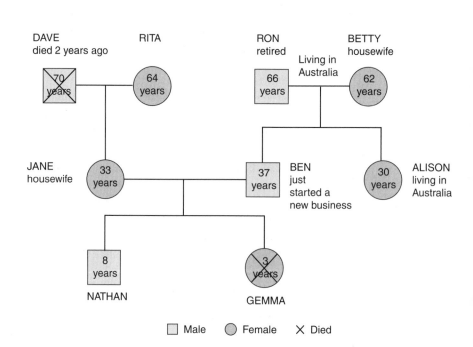

Some of the pain, distress and confusion of parental, sibling and grandparent grief was described in earlier chapters. Therefore, as we emphasised in Chapter 6, nurses and midwives need to be able to listen and, where appropriate, offer information

CONSIDERATIONS FOR PRACTICE WITH BEREAVED FAMILY MEMBERS

and suggestions. These aspects of care should never be underestimated, as they can help to reduce stress and increase the family member's ability to cope. The assessment tool can alert the nurse or midwife to various ways to work with family members. Those outlined in this section are:

- supporting bereaved family members
- maintaining family awareness
- working with the complexity of grieving after sudden child death
- ending follow-up care
- another pregnancy following the death.

Box 8.2 lists key points to consider as strategies to assist family members to cope and help each other.

**Box 8.2
Strategies to assist family members to cope and help each other**

Helping bereaved parents

- help them to acknowledge the pain, loss, isolation and vulnerability that they may be feeling
- encourage them to care for themselves physically because grief is hard work and takes time
- indicate that parents may grieve differently and encourage them, if possible, to find ways to show each other that they care
- remember that parents may find it difficult to make contact with health professionals so make an effort to have continuing contact with them
- ensure that they have an information booklet about the grief of parents, siblings and grandparents
- provide information about postmortems, organising funerals and registering the death
- suggest that they might like to put tokens of remembrance into a memory book or box.

Helping bereaved parents help their children
Do offer information and support to enable the parents to:

- talk honestly and openly with children of all ages about what is happening using clear words such as 'death'
- consider sharing feelings and tears with children
- listen sensitively and carefully
- answer children's questions honestly
- explain activities such as seeing the body or going to the funeral and then offer choices to participate
- show care for the surviving children
- reassure children that they are not responsible for the death
- preserve familiar routine activities and boundaries for expected behaviour

**Box 8.2
Continued**

- appreciate that children will grieve in different ways
- talk about the dead child with surviving children and consider looking at photographs, telling stories, marking the anniversary
- seek advice from health professionals if children become distressed or their behaviour changes
- know about available resources such as facilitated group programmes for bereaved children
- be prepared that children will ask about their sibling's death as they grow older and use new cognitive skills to make sense of what happened
- remember that their children's peers are important to them.

Ensure that parents have written information about sibling grief. Pointers to help parents to support their children are given in Appendix 4.

Helping bereaved grandparents
- acknowledge their bereavement
- encourage them to take care of themselves physically because this is often overlooked
- ensure that they have an information booklet on grandparents' grief
- encourage them to take opportunities to talk about their loss if they want to
- suggest that they might like to put tokens of remembrance in a memory book or box.

Helping bereaved grandparents help the parents
Do offer information and support to encourage them to:

- identify ways in which they can show their support for the parents and siblings – remember the PAL acronym on page 103
- follow the parents' cues to talk about the dead child
- mark the anniversaries for the parents (e.g. with a card, visit or flowers).

SUGGESTIONS FOR COPING WITH BEREAVEMENT

During the course of visits, there are various suggestions that may assist individual family members to use personal and social resources in their grieving. Each person's grief is unique and constructed within their world view, so some suggestions may be useful for some people at some point. To avoid suggestions being perceived as restrictive or prescriptive, we have found it helpful to phrase suggestions with 'I wonder if ...', which is not as direct as 'Have you tried ...?'. This allows an idea to be placed in a space where the family member may choose to pick it up or pass on by. A range of ideas and written materials for parents, siblings and grandparents is available from organisations, websites and books (Appendices 1–6) and some suggestions are given in Box 8.3. These recognise the changes that have happened for

**Box 8.3
Suggestions that
may assist
individual family
members in their
grieving**

■ Appreciating the need for physical self-care to have energy to
  cope with stress (e.g. eating, sleeping and resting).

■ Considering different coping strategies. If someone has predominantly
  loss-oriented coping focus, then they might be encouraged to undertake
  some restoration-oriented activities. This could include achieving small
  goals and activities such as cleaning part of the house or going for a
  daily walk.

■ Appreciating that grief is not a steady trajectory – everyone has 'up'
  and 'down' days.

■ Finding ways to gain new insights about one's own and family
  experience, which might include:
  — exploring grief (such as talking, writing a journal, poems, or
    drawing)
  — relating grief to an image (e.g. a maze, waterfall, storm, journey)
  — reading stories of other bereaved family members or self-help grief
    texts
  — accessing resources via the worldwide web (e.g. chat rooms or
    creating a personal web-page memorial).

■ Creating opportunities to talk to other family members about the dead
  child such as asking, 'What do you remember about [name]?'

■ Creating a memory box/book to hold the tokens of remembrance that
  they treasure of the child's life and death.

■ Protecting tokens of remembrance in case of fire or flood by placing
  copies such as photographs and birth certificates in a location other
  than their home.

■ Preparing for birth or death days by inviting other family members for
  a meal, making a cake, releasing balloons or lighting a candle.

■ Buying an ornament for the Christmas tree each year to symbolise
  the child.

■ Remembering the child publicly by writing words about the child in a
  Remembrance Book. These often exist at maternity and children's
  hospitals, funeral directors, mutual help groups and more recently at
  various sites on the worldwide web.

■ Planning a memorial to the child. This might be a gravestone, a
  bench-seat with plaque or a bequest suited to the age and interests
  of the child. The last might include scholarships, books or music
  equipment for the child's school; playground equipment for the child's
  play centre; or toys for the maternity unit where the baby was born.

■ Commemorating the continuation of life by planting a plant/tree/shrub.
  This might be a dwarf version in a plant pot that can be taken if the
  family move house or it could be planted in the family garden/
  public garden or as part of Plant a Tree scheme managed by the
  Woodland Trust.

Box 8.3
Continued

- Identifying particular symbols that have a meaning associated with the dead child, e.g. a plant, a colour, a scent, an item.
- Creating regular rituals such as gardening a particular area in memory of the child or visiting a special place that is associated with the child.
- Attending mutual help groups or structured grief programmes offered for adults and siblings through bereavement agencies.

the individual and their family. Many of the suggestions may be heard by one family member and then passed on to others.

FAMILY AWARENESS

The death of a child affects both individual family members and the family as a whole. As Jane described in Chapter 5, follow-up care is often focused on the parents, and particularly the mother. However, it is possible for health professionals to consider ways in which other family members are part of the experience of the individual they meet. These might include the following:

- Asking a parent 'How are **you**?' and then asking after other family members 'How is [name]?' This acknowledges the loss of others in the family but also enables parents to talk about family interactions, which may give insights into the grief of other family members.
- Offering to meet other family members (e.g. grandparents, fathers) to answer questions and talk about their experience. This may require arranging a meeting at a time that is outside the normal working hours of some health professionals.
- Making sure that the parents have been given information that can be read by other family members such as grandparents. These may help them to cope and to appreciate the grief of other family members.
- Being alert to other concurrent stressors that may diminish family members' ability to support each other. Sometimes the enormity of a child's death means that the stress of existing illness, or recently moving house, is not recognised as a change that also require coping skills and energy from family members.

When health professionals listen to a bereaved parent, the parent may gain new insights about their own grief and ways to manage family relationships. For example, a mother may share her frustration that her mother will not talk about her feelings. 'Have you talked to your mother about how you feel?' gives a suggestion for her to consider. Or asking, 'Do you think your mother is upset for you but does not know how to help?' may assist the mother to explore why her mother is responding in this way.

Previous family losses may be part of the current bereavement. A nurse or midwife can help to identify the effect that this is having on the family. For example, a mother commented that she felt bewildered at the depth of her mother's grief and abandoned at her mother's lack of support. Talking to the grandmother uncovered the story of her own stillborn child. At that time, the GP had told her husband not to talk about the death because it would help her to recover more quickly. The death of her grandchild brought a range of memories and emotions about her previous loss. The grandmother appreciated the opportunity to talk with the health visitor and decided to follow a suggestion to write her child's name in a Book of Remembrance as a way of remembering their place in the family. It can be important to take time to hear the story of other losses, since they are interwoven into family members' current experience of coping with the death.

RESOURCES OUTSIDE THE FAMILY

As we identified in earlier chapters, bereaved parents and siblings do access support from friends and others outside the family. This includes bereavement agencies, mutual help groups and health professionals. Parents need information about local mutual help groups in case they choose to access these. Mutual help groups can provide a valuable resource for some people by offering a different form of support from that of family and health professionals (Appendices 1 and 2). However, the availability of such support does not absolve health professionals from providing ongoing follow-up care.

Nurses and midwives should also have a current list of support agencies and other sources of support such as clergy, spiritual advisors and community leaders. Some voluntary agencies, local churches and health professionals facilitate support groups for parents and siblings, which may have structured programmes or workshops. These may offer strategies to assist family members cope with, and make sense of, the death. Groups for siblings can enable children to meet other bereaved children. Such an opportunity, to be with children who have had a similar change in their lives, may not otherwise occur in everyday settings such as school or playgroups. Neighbours and friends may also provide support and these should not be overlooked. Several health visitors in Dent's study (2000) arranged to meet neighbours to look at ways in which they could help. This might include encouraging them to drop in for a cup of tea, going shopping with the mother, organising an activity with both parents, helping with the children (e.g. taking them to school, taking them out) or making a casserole for the family.

WORKING WITH THE COMPLEXITY OF GRIEVING AFTER SUDDEN DEATH

Sudden death is likely to preclude saying goodbye; it creates a changed world in which family members may have strong feelings of anger or guilt, which may be related to the nature of the death. The goal of follow-up care is not to take away or ignore such feelings. However, listening to people in pain, distress and despair can be exhausting, which is why nurses and midwives need to have strategies for self care (see Ch. 9). One strategy is to be aware of, and prepared for, some aspects of their distress. It is also important to be aware of indicators of more complex problems that may need access to other professional help.

STRONG FEELINGS IN DISTRESS

The stories in the middle chapters highlight some of the pain, blackness and confusion after sudden child death. We have selected six issues for comment here.

Anger and rage

Although not all bereaved people will feel angry, anger is a common feature. It can be both confusing and difficult to manage because it is not necessarily seen as a socially acceptable part of grief. Anger can be felt towards the deceased because they have left (Worden 1991). While rational thought indicates that the deceased did not choose to go, the feelings of anger at being left or abandoned can remain. Sometimes anger can become directed towards anyone perceived as altering the course of events: this can be self, health professionals, other family members, or God in the bigger picture. Talking about the reasons for feeling anger can offer a way to acknowledge rather than bury the anger. Asking questions such as 'Do you feel angry towards anyone or want to hurt anyone?' may enable people to talk about an emotion that is often perceived as socially unacceptable.

When a child has died violently, some parents may feel extreme anger at the person or agency responsible for the death. This can become rage, with fantasies of violence towards those people perceived to have killed the child (Redmond 1996). Such powerful, unknown images and feelings may be very frightening. Nurses and midwives may be able to acknowledge such feelings and, in doing so, diminish the potential for violent action. Alternatively, the person may find it useful to talk to a counsellor who is skilled at working with survivors of trauma.

Feelings of guilt

As the comments in the earlier chapters indicated, guilt is part of some people's experiences. There is the potential for such feelings to be engendered by others. As Harman (1981, p. 36) described, '*If the bereaved mother does not initially feel guilty she certainly will shortly thereafter by dint of the many "professionals" who repeatedly tell her not to feel guilty.*' Some grieving people feel guilty about imagined or real omissions, such as not having told the deceased how much they were loved or believing that a different decision could have changed the outcome. 'If only, we had not gone home that way he would not have been in the accident.' For parents, guilt can reflect a sense of parental responsibility to 'look after' their child. For a few parents and siblings, feelings of guilt may be entangled with ambivalent feelings about the child when they were alive. Worden (1991, p. 45) described how health professionals might assist.

> Whatever the reasons, most of this guilt is irrational and centers around the circumstances of the death. The counsellor can help here because irrational guilt yields itself up to **reality testing**. If someone says, 'I didn't do enough,' I'll ask, 'What did you do?' and they'll answer, 'I did that.' And then I'll say, 'What else did you do?' 'Well, I did this.' 'What else?' 'Well, I did that.' And then more things will occur to them and they will say, 'I did this, and this, and this.' After a while they will come to the conclusion, 'Maybe I did all I could do under the circumstances'.

Sometimes guilt arises because of real culpability in the death, such as driving the car in which the child died. Because of the challenge that this may present to a family member, health professionals might work with the family member to access other resources such as an experienced counsellor.

The cause of death

The cause of a child's death is not always identified even after postmortem. This can leave parents permanently wondering why their child died. In some circumstances, such as sudden infant death syndrome (SIDS), they may wonder whether it might happen again with another child. During follow-up visits, health professionals can listen to parents as they seek an answer. It may be necessary to organise a further appointment with relevant professionals such as a paediatrician or obstetrician, since information discussed at an appointment 6 weeks after the death may not be fully remembered. Even when the cause of death is known, many parents have outstanding questions from the postmortem. Dent et al (1996) found that over a fifth of parents (n = 67) in their study did not understand the postmortem findings and a small number were not able to ask questions at the time. An appointment may need to be organised with a paediatrician or pathologist (preferably with a paediatric focus) who can provide time to answer any questions that the parents might have.

Parents' questions are an attempt to understand and locate the death within existing knowledge about the world. Questions may include 'What happened?' 'Who was there?' 'Why did it happen?' 'Does it happen often?' 'Could it have been prevented?' 'Will it happen again?' The last may be a central question to families who have experienced miscarriage or death of a baby and are considering future pregnancies. Again, the nurse or midwife may be able to answer some questions, clarify some points and arrange for the parents to meet a paediatrician or obstetrician.

Violent death

Violent death can occur as a result of vehicle crash, a plane crash, murder or a bombing. Deaths, such as murder, can bring a sense of stigma for the survivors, often leading to a lack of social support (Redmond 1996). Therefore, it is extremely important that support is available from health professionals. In addition, if a person or agency is culpable for the death, the parents' grief may be entangled for years awaiting the outcome of criminal proceedings. In a few instances, the person charged with responsibility for the child's death may also be a member of the child's family. This can create enormous stress for other family members, who face multiple losses within the changed family world. To be able to support bereaved families involved with the judicial system requires health professionals to have some understanding of the criminal justice system and to appreciate the emotional and financial costs that may overtake the grief of bereaved families (Lord 1996, Redmond 1996). However, Dent (2000) found that health professionals were not involved in the few cases analysed where legal proceedings were being taken. This raises the issue of provision of follow-up care. Who assists such families, who may be in great need of support?

Nurses and midwives also need to consider the language used by family members to describe the violent death. Family members may feel that '*died*' is too passive whereas '*killed*' indicates that '*life was taken, not simply lost*' (Lord 1996, p. 33). Similarly, '*crash*' can reflect that it is '*somebody's fault*' (Lord 1996, p. 32) in contrast to 'accident'.

Suicide

Many of the issues such as guilt, stigmatisation and involvement of the judicial system described under violent death are pertinent to families who are survivors of suicide. As we noted before, acknowledgement by, and ongoing contact with, a health professional is a central part of follow-up care. Stillion (1996), citing van der Wal, noted that bereavement after suicide differs from other deaths in various respects: family members are more likely to deny the cause of death, search for a motive and have feelings of rejection. This is illustrated in some of the comments from parents in Chapter 3. Family members may require specialist counselling to enable them to cope with the meaning that the death holds in their lives.

Difficult deaths

The comments in Chapters 3–5 illustrate that many parents, siblings and grandparents find ways over the years to continue with activities, relationships and decisions while living with the experience of the sudden death of a child. Parkes (2001), too, noted that many people go through bereavement without counselling or specialist support; their existing social and personal resources are sufficient. Other people have difficulty with their grief. A few may experience serious physical or mental ill-health unless additional resources are made available (Parkes 2001). As we noted above, the sudden death of a child may potentially be a 'difficult' death to grieve and there may be a lack of social and cultural resources to assist individuals (Riches & Dawson 2000). Nurses and midwives can assist such individuals to recognise their distress, discomfort or difficulty in coping and to access other resources, such as professionals whose specialty is working with the bereaved.

ACCESSING RESOURCES OFFERED BY OTHER PROFESSIONALS

When might a family member need additional resources beyond the support of family, friends, mutual help groups and a nurse or midwife? Nurses and midwives can use a range of information to make this assessment **with** a family member. The following points can help to guide discussions and assessment.

Listen to individual family members. They know themselves better than anyone else, many identifying difficulties with their grief. With someone to listen, possible sources of support may be explored. They may decide that support from a professional, such as a counsellor, may be appropriate.

Listen to other family members. They know each other. They may identify when a family member is having difficulty continuing with everyday activities. They may also feel that they no longer know how to help. The health professional can encourage family members to talk together, assisting them to identify resources, such as counselling.

Recognise the need for ongoing assessment and the limitation of information based on one meeting. All people have 'good' and 'bad' days. Grief generally changes over time, moving from acute distress to ways of coping. While the rate of movement may be imperceptible at times, meeting family members on several occasions will enable health professionals to assess whether grief is changing. Is the pain less intense? Are there oscillations between feelings and everyday activities? Are there moments when life is not as black? Is the person caring for themselves physically? Are they providing any necessary physical care for children in the family? Are they, or children in the family, at risk of ill-health or injury as a result of the ways in which they are responding to the death?

Remember the importance of context as part of assessment. What are the concurrent stressors? What is the individual's coping style? How much available social support is there?

Be sensitive to indicators of other problems. The ways in which an individual is talking or behaving might indicate that there may be:

- particular stresses arising because of the type of death (see earlier discussion)
- particular stresses arising from a traumatic death (Appendix 12)
- grieving that might be viewed as complicated (Appendix 12)
- an individual having suicidal thoughts (see Appendix 12).

The situation may also occur where a health professional finds working with some family members 'difficult'. This can reflect uncertainty and lack of confidence in practice, particularly when faced with some of the complexities of bereavement following sudden death of a child. In such an instance, the health professional needs to recognise their responsibility to provide follow-up care that offers assistance to family members. If they doubt their ability to do so, or have concerns about the parent's well-being, they might negotiate with the family member to revisit with another colleague who has experience working with bereaved families. This has the potential then to support the family and to assist the health professional to access necessary care for the family member. In some situations, this model of joint visiting may assist in mentoring new practitioners while they gain confidence to work with bereaved families.

A family member may choose to talk to another professional in detail about their experience, or the identified nurse or midwife may have concerns about the well-being of an individual. In either instance, the nurse or midwife might begin by discussing the situation with the GP involved with the family. The discussion can explore options for referral, which, depending on the locality and the availability of funding, might include a nurse or doctor working in the field of mental health, a counsellor or a therapist. Any referral should be made with the consent of the individual concerned. The suggestion of 'counselling' or other professional resources may have different meanings to different family members. Some may be unwilling to access such services, either because it is seen as a sign of weakness and not coping (Stewart 1988) or because it is unknown and outside their frame of reference. Hindmarch (2000, p. 166) proposed the following indicators for people who may find such services useful:

- *low self esteem*
- *persistent suicidal feelings*
- *breakdown of relationships*
- *multiple or coincidental losses*
- *traumatic circumstances surrounding the death.*

She also noted that resources, such as counselling, might be of maximum use in the longer term and not in the first few days and weeks following a death.

Some family members who are uncertain about seeking assistance may appreciate the company of a familiar nurse or midwife when meeting an unfamiliar professional. Nurses and midwives already involved in follow-up can continue to keep in contact with the family and work as a member of the team alongside another professional.

ENDING FOLLOW-UP BEREAVEMENT CARE

The ending of follow-up care is as important as the initial visit. There is no fixed time to end bereavement follow-up. For a number of families, this may be after the first anniversary. The following questions may help the health professional and the parent to realise that support is no longer necessary:

- can they talk about the dead child without being engulfed in emotion?
- how do they describe their grief?
- do they feel that their grief has changed over time?
- how did they cope with and feel about meaningful dates such as 6 months and 12 months after the death?
- what strategies have they learnt to manage painful feelings?
- what insights do they have about other family members' grief?
- how would they describe their relationships with other family members since the death?
- how do they feel about life in general?
- do they have times of feeling confident and looking forward to events?
- do they care for themselves and other family members physically?

In many instances, the relationship between the health professional and family member(s) will continue, but the purpose of visits will change focus. For example, a health visitor may cease to concentrate on bereavement follow-up and future visits will centre on health promotion and well-child assessment of surviving siblings. Some family members mark the ending as a special occasion, by giving a card, or a drawing made by other siblings, to the health professional.

ANOTHER PREGNANCY FOLLOWING THE DEATH

Some parents will consider having future children soon after the death, particularly when a miscarriage has occurred. Parents may have different reasons for wanting a child. Parents' decisions about whether and when to have a child are influenced by reasons such as:

- age and fertility of the parents
- whether the family is perceived as complete
- likelihood of recurrence of death, e.g. if previous child died of a genetic condition
- expectations of other family members.

Interpretation of articles about a 'replacement child', such as Cain and Cain (1964) and Poznanski (1972) may have contributed to the advice given to some parents to wait a year and take time to grieve before having another child. However, some of the perspectives presented in Chapter 3 indicate that parental bereavement is life-long and begs the question 'When is a 'good' time to have another child?' Rose described her decision to leave the outcome to God (p. 49). Grout and Romanoff (2000) undertook a study with 10 parents who had experienced the death of a baby and then had a subsequent child, aged 3–5 years at the time of the research. They found that many parents found ways to maintain a place for the dead child in the family. Some parents replaced the loss of **a** child but not necessarily **the** child who had died. The findings reaffirm the earlier discussion about the diverse meanings that individuals create about their bereavement. This indicates that definitive advice on the timing of another pregnancy may not suit all parents. Therefore, it would seem important to support parents in making choices that are congruent with their own beliefs and feelings. Health professionals might suggest waiting at least 3 months after the death to avoid the birth being around the same time of year as the death. Pregnancy, the birth and the following weeks can prove challenging and distressing for parents and other family members. As Rose described in Chapter 5, sudden death of a child can bring a sense of vulnerability and uncertainty about life that permeates the experience of another pregnancy.

CARE DURING A SUBSEQUENT PREGNANCY

The following points may be helpful when caring for families during a pregnancy following the death of a baby. They may also be useful for parents who have experienced the death of an older child and who may have lost some of their confidence in their ability to be parents.

Antenatally and during labour

Help needs to be tailored to the situation of the previous child death:

- offer a chance to review questions about the child's death
- ensure health professionals involved in the care are aware of the child's death and provide opportunities for the parents to talk
- offer any relevant tests and care that might prevent recurrence of another sudden death during pregnancy or labour (e.g. placental insufficiency, rhesus iso-immunisation)
- offer contact details of any mutual help groups or individuals who are able to provide information and support based on experience of having another child.

Postnatal care

Parents may need particular reassurance about the health of their baby regardless of the circumstances of their previous loss:

- offer opportunities for physical examination of the baby by a paediatrician
- offer sufficient support to sustain parents' self-confidence to care for a young baby (e.g. additional home visits, 24 hour contact number).

It can also be useful to offer parents information on childcare practices that may promote parents' sense of confidence and help to reduce the risk of any future deaths. Information might include the following:

- ways to protect babies from accidents, infection and cot death (e.g. discuss using accompanying information booklet of BabyZone, published in 2003, available from FSID from www.sids.org.uk)
- cardiopulmonary resuscitation training in parent-craft classes or at St John's Ambulance.

Thoughts of the dead child are often in the parents' minds; the new baby may elicit visual memories of the dead child. Sometimes family and friends do not mention the dead child because of concerns about introducing sadness at a time of celebration. After the birth, health professionals might acknowledge to parents the continuing place of the child who died. This could be a comment such as:

- 'Does this baby look like [name]?'
- 'This baby will enjoy looking at the photos of [name] when older'.

After the death of a baby or recurrent miscarriages, there are specialist support services available for families in some localities. This generally involves obstetricians, paediatricians, GPs, midwives and health visitors working to support families. An example is the Care of the Next Infant (CONI) programme scheme supported by the Foundation for Sudden Infant Death. Established during the late

1980s in different areas of the UK, it offers families the opportunity for weekly home visits from their health visitor with strategies such as using a symptom chart and apnoea monitor (see www.sids.org.uk).

SUMMARY

Supporting bereaved families and being allowed into parts of their lives at a time of change and tragedy is a privilege. Box 8.4 lists some of the skills needed for caring for bereaved families over time based on the acronym COMPASSION (see the similar skill list for the period immediately surrounding a death in Box 7.1).

Providing such support is also demanding and stressful for the health professional. He or she needs to be able to assess the change in level of support needed with time and to be aware of subsequent problems that may need referring for other professional help. The next chapter considers how health professionals can cope with the challenges that such work can bring.

SUMMARY POINTS

- All families whose child has died suddenly should be offered the opportunity to have follow-up support by a health professional.
- Some family members have an extensive range of personal and social resources to help them to cope with the death and may not desire follow-up.
- Health professionals are one of a range of social resources that are available to family members.
- Follow-up can include an assessment of the stressors or concerns identified by the parents so that health professionals can plan care to assist the parents.
- While parents, and often the mother, are the main point of contact, it is important to be aware of how other family members are coping with the death.
- For a range of reasons, some family members experience difficulties. Nurses and midwives need to be aware of the extent of their skills and enable family members to access other professionals when appropriate.
- COMPASSION provides an acronym for considerations in practice that are relevant to continuing follow-up care (see Box 8.4).
- Having another baby after a child has died can be a difficult time for parents and other family members; health professionals can help families to cope by being aware of their concerns and offering extra resources.

Box 8.4   Caring for bereaved families over time

C are and compassion are key elements. Do you have these qualities?

O ffer yourself as a fellow-human being, listening carefully and actively. Remember your body language will convey what you are thinking.

M essage of grief. Recognise that the pain of grief cannot be taken away; there are no instant solutions.

P lan family care with the parents to include surviving children and grandparents, where appropriate.

A rrange a case conference, if appropriate, with all professionals involved with the death to assess and plan future care of the family.

S eek help, if possible, if you feel overwhelmed or out of your depth. Who can you go and talk to?

S upervision or workplace support should be available to you. Do you have sufficient time to debrief and learn from each situation?

I dentify stressors in the family, as perceived by the parents at each visit and work to reduce these whenever possible.

O ffer regular visits and ensure that family members know where to contact voluntary bereavement agencies and mutual help groups.

N ever make assumptions about the experience of bereaved family members. Avoid platitudes such as 'I know just how you feel'.

This page may be photocopied.
We would appreciate acknowledgement to Dent and Stewart (2003) *Sudden death in childhood: support for the bereaved family.* Elsevier Science, Edinburgh

REFERENCES

Cain AC, Cain BS 1964 On replacing a child. Journal of the American Academy of Child Psychiatry 3: 443–456

de Montigny F, Beaudet L, Dumas L 1999 A baby has died: the impact of perinatal loss on family social networks. Journal of Obstetric, Gynaecology and Neonatal Nursing 28: 151–155

Dent A 2000 Support for families whose child dies suddenly from accident or illness. PhD thesis, School of Policy Studies, University of Bristol, UK

Dent A 2002 Family support after sudden child death. Community Practitioner 75: 469–473

Dent A, Condon L, Fleming P et al 1996 A study of bereavement care after sudden and unexpected death. Archives of Disease in Childhood 74: 522–526

Finlay I, Dallimore D 1991 Your child is dead. British Medical Journal 302: 1524–1525

Gaines J, Arnold J, Jessop DJ et al 1996 Home visits to bereaved families subsequent to sudden infant death: a demonstration project. Journal of Sudden Death Syndrome and Infant Mortality 1: 33–45

Grout LA, Romanoff BD 2000 The myth of the replacement child: parents' stories and practices after perinatal death. Death Studies 24: 93–113

Harman W 1981 Death of my baby. British Medical Journal 282: 35–37

Hindmarch C 2000 On the death of a child, 2nd edn. Radcliffe Medical Press, Oxford

Lazarus RS, Folkman S 1984 Stress, appraisal and coping. Springer-Verlag, New York

Lindsey B, Elsegood J (eds) 1996 Working with children in grief and loss. Baillière Tindall, London

Lord JH 1996 America's number one killer: vehicular crashes. In: Doka K (ed) Living with grief after sudden loss. Taylor & Francis, Philadelphia, PA, p 25–41

Malacrida C 1998 Mourning the dreams. Qual Institute Press, University of Alberta, Edmonton, Alberta

Moulder C 2001 Miscarriage: women's experiences and needs, 2nd edn. Routledge, London

Murray J 1993 An ache in their hearts. University of Queensland, Brisbane, Australia

Parkes C 2001 A historical overview of the scientific study of bereavement. In: Stroebe M, Hansson R, Stroebe W et al (eds) Handbook of bereavement research. American Psychological Association, Washington, DC, p 25–45

Poznanski E 1972 The 'replacement child': a saga of unresolved parental grief. Behavioural Pediatrics 81: 1190–1193

Rando T 1986a The unique issues and impact of the death of a child. In: Rando T (ed) Parental loss of a child. Research Press, Champaign IL, p 3–44

Rando T 1986b Parental bereavement: an exception to the general conceptualisations of mourning. In: Rando T (ed) Parental loss of a child. Research Press, Champaign IL, p 45–58

Rando T 1986c Individual and couples treatment following the death of a child. In: Rando T (ed) Parental loss of a child. Research Press, Champaign IL, p 341–413

Rando T 1993 Treatment of complicated mourning. Research Press, Champaign, IL

Rando T 1996 Complications in mourning traumatic death. In: Doka K (ed) Living with grief after sudden loss. Taylor & Francis, Philadelphia, PA, p 139–159

Raphael B 1984 The anatomy of bereavement, 3rd edn. Unwin Hyman, London

Redmond L 1996 Sudden violent death. In: Doka K (ed) Living with grief after sudden loss. Taylor & Francis, Philadelphia, PA, p 53–73

Riches G, Dawson P 1996a 'An intimate loneliness': evaluating the impact of a child's death on parental self-identity and marital relationships. Journal of Family Therapy 18: 1–22

Riches G, Dawson P 1996b Communities of feeling: the culture of bereaved families. Mortality 1: 143–161

Riches G, Dawson P 2000 An intimate loneliness: supporting bereaved parents and siblings. Open University Press, Buckingham, UK

Stewart M 1988 The anguish of being in need. Bereavement Care 7: 17–18

Stillion JM 1996 Survivors of suicide. In: Doka K (ed) Living with grief and loss. Taylor & Francis, Philadelphia, PA, p 41–53

Stroebe M, Schut H 2001 Meaning making in the dual process of coping with bereavement. In: Neimeyer R (ed) Meaning reconstruction and the experience of loss. American Psychological Association, Washington, DC, p 55–75

Stroebe M, Stroebe W, Hansson R (eds) 1993 Handbook of bereavement: theory, research and intervention. Cambridge University Press, New York

Worden JW 1983 Grief counselling and grief therapy. Tavistock, London

Worden JW 1991 Grief counselling and grief therapy, 2nd edn. Routledge, London

USEFUL SOURCES FOR NURSES AND MIDWIVES

Hindmarch C 2000 On the death of a child 2nd edn. Radcliffe Medical Press, Oxford

Kohner N, Henley A 2001 When a baby dies, 2nd edn. Routledge, London

Moulder C 2001 Miscarriage: women's experiences and needs, 2nd edn. Routledge, London

Riches G, Dawson P 2000 Intimate loneliness: supporting bereaved parents and siblings. Open University Press, Buckingham, UK

Warland J 2000 The midwife and the bereaved family. Ausmed, Ascot Vale, Australia

Wright B 1996 Sudden death 2nd edn. Churchill Livingstone, London

Stress and loss: resources for health professionals

> *The fact that we deal with people who are vulnerable makes us vulnerable too, and if we are to remain truly human when coping with our own difficulties and those of other people, then we need to be supported for our own good and the good of those for whom we care.*
>
> Tschudin 1987

INTRODUCTION

And so we come to the last chapter of our book. In previous chapters, we have considered the ways in which health professionals might support bereaved family members after the sudden death of a child. This chapter is specifically about health professionals, without whom the care described in the other chapters could not be offered. What is their experience of caring for bereaved families? How do they cope with the emotional demands? How can they be supported to continue with this valuable work? In previous chapters, we have written as the authors offering considerations for practice. In this chapter, we place ourselves alongside all health professionals working in this challenging area of practice and use 'we' to include ourselves and the reader.

THE EXPERIENCES OF HEALTH PROFESSIONALS

CARE FOR OURSELVES

One of the challenges we faced, as authors, was what to include in this chapter. We wondered if the subject of care for ourselves had become 'old hat'. It is included in a range of textbooks and is part of preregistration education and postregistration workshops and programmes. Yet in workshops, we meet health professionals who 'know' about strategies for self-care and but do not practise these. Why? People reply with a range of reasons including: tiredness, lack of time, 'it won't change anything', and lack of organisational support in the form of time or support resources. It seems that there is a danger that care for ourselves becomes an accepted rhetoric that is reflected neither in personal practice nor in the cultural and social contexts within which we work. Many professionals desire knowledge to be able to work in practice with grieving families, but that same knowledge has relevance for our own well-being. It is important to recognise that we are people first and health professionals second. Like the family members we support, we are individuals and as such are likely to be part of a family that brings joys, difficulties and stresses to our lives. We are also part of the wider social community in which we live. Therefore, we bring to the workplace our unique contribution, which includes our past personal and professional experiences. At times, we may have to juggle pressures at home and at work. We are not superhuman; we are vulnerable beings as Tschudin (1987) reminded us at the beginning of the chapter. We will have many pressures on our time and our skills, but supporting families after sudden child death is probably one of the most demanding and stressful. When we give a lot of ourselves, we need to be replenished. If we want to be effective helpers, we need to be effective people first, and look for support, even demand it, because without support for ourselves, we cannot realistically support bereaved families.

SUPPORTING FAMILIES

We begin by looking at what health professionals feel about supporting families. These are some of the comments that professionals in practice have made (Dent et al 1996, Dent 2000).

I think supporting parents who have lost a child is one of the hardest jobs we are expected to do and one [for] which we are hugely ill-prepared and consequently dread.

The sudden death of a child is a highly stressful event for all involved, including the family's health visitor.

In the face of such a loss to the family, I felt I had little comfort to offer. I have children of my own and felt their vulnerability more intensely. 'There but for the grace of God go I.'

I was trying to do the right thing for the family, which is not necessarily what I considered to be appropriate to my own thoughts and feelings.

Each comment carries an individual message but all demonstrate the burden of supporting bereaved families.

Just as bereaved family members are unique. so too are health professionals. Each will perceive stress differently and this may vary at different times in their lives. As Fontana (1990, p. 61) noted, it is the combination of *'what it is in us, that makes us perceive things as stressful or not, and what it is in us that determines whether we can handle this stress or not'*. Therefore, at any given time, what is 'stressful' to one health professional may not be for another. Consequently, like working in practice with family members, we cannot offer generalised solutions or give pointers for self-care to suit **all** health professionals. However, we can consider the stressors that health professionals may encounter when supporting a family after sudden death of a child.

CHALLENGES OF CARING FOR GRIEVING FAMILIES

As we discussed in Chapter 6, health professionals can be challenged for various reasons in their practice. These are a few examples of challenges that may become stressors.

The paradox of being involved while maintaining detachment. As Tschudin (1987) described at the beginning of this chapter, health professionals face a constant paradox: that of being involved in people's lives, engaging in care with compassion or empathy and then finding a way to move on and care for the next person and their family.

Doubts about actions. When resuscitation or treatment preceded the death, a health professional may wonder whether they did everything that could be done to save life. Faced with an angry grieving parent who says it is the 'midwife's fault' their baby died, such thoughts may be intensified.

Death as the antithesis of the birth. If practice is constructed as enabling people to live, death may represent a failure. The intensive care environment has been called 'a combat zone' (Wagner & Higdon 1996, p. 20); this could equally apply to accident and emergency care. In contrast, midwifery practice has a focus on the creation of life, which means that death is the antithesis of the expected outcome of pregnancy and labour.

Personal sense of mortality. The death of another person and the grief of family members can touch a professional's personal sense of mortality. They can generate questions such as: 'What is the purpose of life?' 'What am I doing here?' 'Why do children die?'

Reminders of personal losses. Working with angry, upset and grieving people can trigger reminders of a health professional's personal losses, such as relationships that ended and the hurt that has not gone away.

Ethical dilemmas.   Some situations pose ethical dilemmas. A family's decision to withdraw life-support may conflict with a professional's personal beliefs about preservation of life.

The shock of suddenness.   The suddenness of death can be a shock for health professionals as well as for family members.

We come into our professional work with a wide range of motives, attitudes and ambitions. Sometimes the ideals and expectations of our earlier vocation become jaded because of particular situations, pressure of work, changes in an employing organisation and other concurrent life stresses. Consider the two quotes below that illustrate a sense of continuing stress (Montgomery 1993, pp. 108 and 109, respectively).

> *Each time I let someone into my heart, when they die, it's just like I close off even more. It's just like, OK, I'm going to do what I have to do.*

> *It's like I can see [the families] wanting to feel like somebody cares, but they just don't understand. [I've] seen this three or four times a month for 10 years, you don't have it to care. I mean – I don't mean that you don't care, but ... it's kind of like you close off a certain part of yourself. You have nothing to give these people other than you try to be nice.*

CONSEQUENCES OF STRESS

Continuing stress may both become a risk to professional practice and affect all aspects of personal well-being, including:

- physical changes such as fatigue, energy loss, digestive disturbances, difficulty sleeping, loss of appetite, sleep disturbances
- cognitive changes such as lack of concentration, difficulty remembering information, becoming overconfident or inflexible
- emotional changes such as feeling irritable, tearful, angry, hopeless or powerless.

Stress may appear as cynicism, withdrawal into procedures and protocols or low morale (Capewell & Beattie 1996). Burnout, as a consequence of stress, has received continuing attention. As Freudenberger (1974, p. 159) noted, there is an aptness in the use of this term which means '*to fail, wear out, or become exhausted by making excessive demands on energy, strength or resources*'. A midwife described her experience of prolonged stress in practice.

> *I was like an empty reservoir, the rains never came and the water kept on being taken out. The staffing levels meant I was constantly caring for several women in labour at the same time. At times when a baby died, it took the little energy that I had to show the care that I wanted to give, and that I thought they deserved. There was never a chance to stop and think; each day seemed hard and I forgot small things like why I had gone to the office to get something. Then one day I snapped at a colleague. And I thought, 'This isn't me, what is happening?'*

Recently, Figley (1995) has written about 'compassion fatigue', a secondary traumatic stress disorder occurring when professionals care for people experiencing trauma. While contributors to Figley's book have tended to focus on first responders and therapists, it has relevance for nurses and midwives. As we noted in Chapter 8, a number of unexpected deaths are traumatic deaths for surviving family members, who are supported by health professionals in accident and emergency and primary health care. While stress may play a part in caring for bereaved families, grief also needs consideration.

HEALTH PROFESSIONALS AS GRIEVERS?

Health professionals may have various reasons to grieve. Papadatou (2000) recently proposed a model of health professionals' grief. She integrated theoretical writings with her own experience as a clinical psychologist, combined with the experiences of 63 nurses. The nurses worked with children in oncology or intensive care settings in Greece and Hong Kong, so her model is based on both sudden and anticipated deaths. She suggested that professionals may face various losses (Papadatou 2000, pp. 62–63):

- *loss of a close relationship with a particular patient*
- *loss due to professional's identification with the pain of family members*
- *loss of one's unmet goals and expectations and one's professional self-image and role*
- *losses related to one's personal system of beliefs and assumptions about life*
- *past unresolved losses or anticipated future losses*
- *the death of self.*

Losses vary according to factors such as the relationship with a child and their family, personal experiences, and professional identity. For example, a nurse working in accident and emergency may not identify a personal loss of a close relationship when a child arrives dead. The nurse may, however, feel a loss of professional self-image and role by being a member of a team that was unable to resuscitate a child. Another nursing colleague, involved in the same situation, may feel the loss of certainty in life. By comparison, the health visitor, who has seen the child and family regularly over several years, may feel a personal loss of the child she has watched growing up.

In Chapter 2, we discussed the dual process model of Stroebe and Schut (1999, 2001), which suggested that grieving people oscillate between loss- and restoration-oriented coping. Papadatou (2000, p. 66) also proposed that health professionals fluctuate between a '*focus on the loss*' to '*a movement away*' from it. The first may produce a wide range of reactions, including:

- crying
- feeling angry and/or guilty
- sharing the experience with others.

Whereas, '*movement away*' involves:

- '*shutting out feelings*' (I must be strong, I must control my grief because I wear a uniform)
- '*avoidance of contact*' with the family by being physically absent or creating in oneself a sense of not being present
- '*retreating to practical tasks*'.

If stress and loss is part of working practice, how do health professionals cope with it?

RECOGNISING AND ACKNOWLEDGING STRESS OR LOSS

A range of reasons such as high workloads, patient acuity and workplace beliefs that 'carers just cope and keep on going', can mean that we do not recognise the stress and loss experienced in the workplace. Do we need to? Arguably, only if there are changes to our well-being, otherwise an event is not a stressor or a loss. Reflection on practice and discussions with other people can help to acknowledge any stresses and losses that make practice uncomfortable. Recognition and acknowledgement of stresses and losses may be privately to oneself or they may be shared with others. It may, but does not always, mean owning and expressing emotions. We have met some health professionals who have found it useful to describe powerful emotions arising from their work such as anger, fear, frustration and sadness. Just as bereaved family members find such emotions intense and overwhelming, so can health professionals. We have also met health professionals who have not wanted to talk about their feelings but have found it useful to identify the stressors or losses that were associated with their experiences such as tiredness, insomnia and losing or gaining weight. We each need to assess these factors for ourselves.

- How do you perceive stress and loss? Are they part of your working life?
- What strategies or processes do you use to live with stress and loss in your working life?

RESOURCES: MAINTAINING AND SUSTAINING OURSELVES

To prevent and respond to stress and loss, we potentially have the same personal, social and cultural resources as bereaved family members. This was described by Riches and Dawson (2000) in the context of grieving, see page 39. Some of the resources listed in Appendix 8 offer further ideas for self-care.

PERSONAL RESOURCES

As we discussed in the earlier chapters, personal resources within each of us are central to managing stress, crisis, loss and grief in our working practice. These include beliefs, values, previous experiences and existing coping strategies to manage situations of stress and loss. There are many ways of dealing with stress so the following section presents only a few. Activities involve care of oneself as a physical, cognitive, emotional, social and spiritual being. Coping with death and the pain of bereavement means that we may have to reconnect with ourselves and allow investment in life and living. We may need to remind ourselves that our professional practice is only one part of ourselves.

General physical and psychological care

Some of the activities we have listed may not appeal to everyone. However, all are worth considering, particularly if we have a sense of discomfort and difficulty with stress.

Affirming a sense of one-self.   If health professionals' business is about promoting health and well-being of others, then we have a responsibility towards ourselves.

Making choices about our diet.   Is our diet balanced? Is there any merit in short-term supplements such as the vitamin B series, which may become depleted during prolonged stress. Do we drink water regularly each day?

Making choices about lifestyle.   Do we have enough time to rest? What assists and hinders sleeping? Is some form of regular exercise a part of our day?

Using relaxation.   The physical tensions created by stress can be offset by relaxation, which allow a focus back to a sense of self. We often forget to breathe properly when stressed. Breathing in through the nose, filling up the abdomen like a balloon and then breathing out slowly can help muscles to relax.

Meditation.   This may help us focus attention away from stress or loss to concentrate on other aspects of life.

Humour.   Cultivating a sense of humour can help us to maintain a sense of perspective about life.

A positive life view.   Cultivating a positive view of life may balance the painful experiences that we meet in practice.

Relaxing activities.   Finding activities that are about 'being in the moment' and not about doing things. It might be meditation, listening to music or sitting on a beach.

Reaffirming a sense of self.   Expand a sense of self in the world, perhaps by exploring the aesthetics of life through art, gardening, reading, films or music.

Exploring one's own spirituality.   Recognise and exploring one's own spirituality whether as a member of a religious or spiritual group or through other media such as yoga.

Spiritual and philosophical resources

The most significant individual quality that can help carers create positive meaning when dealing with stress and exposure to death is a philosophical or spiritual understanding. Sometimes it is hard to find a meaning about a child's death. Individuals find their own way to make sense of experiences as two nurses described (Montgomery 1993, pp. 114 and 115, respectively).

I have many images of patients I've lost. They're real for me, they're spirits ... they pass life on to me. I am instructed to live because they were not able to ... I have a responsibility to them who died so young ... to live life more fully, to be really aware of what life is ... We have a responsibility to be all that we can be.

So long as you remember people, they never die ... we sometimes avoid being attached to people in this business because we are afraid of the pain. But there is a lesson to be learnt from that, and it isn't just pain we should be looking at ... and sometimes you can't have one without the other. And I'm not tearful because I'm sad, that's not it at all. Sometimes I think tears are a sign of fullness, and when you overflow, you overflow.

Reflection

Reflection in, and on, practice can enable us to use our personal resources to gain new insights and meanings about experiences that may cause stress or loss.

Each day at work and at home, we encounter new situations, ideas and changes in our own physical and emotional health. These can act as stressors or offer new perspectives to integrate into our assumptive world. Reflection about practice and life outside work offers an opportunity to appreciate aspects of ourselves in relation to the world. Reflection may help to identify stressors, acknowledge losses, explore ways of finding a meaning and recognise the ways that beliefs can shape practice. For the purposes of this chapter, we have used Taylor's work (2000) as a framework since many health professionals find it useful. Taylor (2000, p. 3) offered the following definition:

reflection means the throwing back of thoughts and memories, in cognitive acts such as thinking, contemplation, meditation and any other form of attentive consideration, in order to make sense of them, and to make contextually appropriate changes if they are required.

Methods for reflection

A journal of stories is often associated with the notion of reflective practice. However, many colleagues are unwilling to do this for a range of reasons including time, unfamiliarity with the process and having difficulty writing about their experiences. Taylor (2000) noted that other creative activities such as painting, dance, music, poetry, quilting, videotaping or singing can also be a means for reflection. Williams and Lowe (2001) proposed that mind maps provide an alternative to journals and included an example from a situation in practice where a child died. While reflection may be a private process, it also occurs during conversations with other people. Finding opportunities to tell our story to others serves a similar process to the role that we take with those bereaved family members who want to talk about their experience. For health professionals, such opportunities can be formalised as part of attending clinical supervision sessions or a support group.

Process of reflection

The aim of reflection is to uncover knowledge that may not be apparent using trigger questions such as 'How?' 'What?' 'Why?' 'Who?' These are often the questions that health professionals ask bereaved family members to gain a 'picture' of their grief and to assist them in finding new perspectives for themselves. As a beginning to reflection, Taylor (2000, p. 56) proposed identifying a situation that went well in practice and asking the following questions:

- *what went well?*
- *why did it go well?*
- *where did it happen?*
- *who was involved?*
- *how were you involved?*
- *what did you do?*
- *why did you do what you did?*
- *what were you thinking about at the time?*
- *what do you think about it now?*

If health professionals feel uncertain about how to use reflection as a strategy, then it is worth remembering that reflection is part of our everyday lives. Many people use reflective skills and questions similar to those listed above when commenting on a conversation or wondering why something has happened.

SOCIAL RESOURCES

As health professionals, and as individuals, we all have interactions with people such as family members, friends, work colleagues, acquaintances and other professionals. Their expectations, beliefs and behaviours can shape our experience of living with stress or loss. In this section, we have focused on social resources from family, friends and the workplace.

Family and friends

Our family and friends are often desired sources of support. They are familiar, they generally care and they are often accessible. They have the potential to offer an informal debriefing of general feelings about the day, by listening and asking questions. However, our desire to talk is often constrained by requirements to maintain confidentiality of information. This may mean that we cannot discuss some situations with family members. Even when it is possible to share unidentifiable aspects of work experiences, some health professionals, like family members, find that family and friends cannot offer the support they want. A nurse working in the neonatal intensive care unit said '*I want to talk to my partner about things that upset me in practice, and he asks about my day. But when I start talking about it, he quickly turns the conversation to what we are going to have for tea or who is going to collect the children from school.*' As she identified, there may be a range of reasons why he did not want to listen, which include having had a difficult day himself, being unable to identify with her work situation, not having a strategy himself for reflecting on situations and not knowing how to respond to her distress. Other health professionals find family and friends may listen but offer comments or advice that are not helpful. This can arise because of lack of knowledge of the practice context, or the particular situation, which cannot be disclosed because of confidentiality. Occasionally, there might be the comment 'I couldn't do what you do – dealing with all that death and you just keep on going'. This implies that the health professional is almost non-human and does not offer acknowledgement of their stress or pain. Consequently, for a range of reasons, the opportunity to receive support from friends and family about workplace experiences may be limited or even frustrating. This means that work colleagues may become a *'surrogate family'* (Papadatou 2000, p. 74) and form a pivotal social resource to help individuals to cope.

Informal support from workplace colleagues

Social resources in the workplace may be both structured and unstructured. Peer support is probably the most common type of informal support that is easily available, both in hospitals and in the community. Dent (2000) found that health visitors received the greatest support from colleagues who listened to, and were there for, each other. Such support includes:

- role-modelling strategies for coping with stressors or losses such as death
- sharing ideas and information that assist an individual to cope
- asking 'How are you?' and wanting to hear the answer
- listening and sometimes offering thoughts to individuals as they seek to reflect on, and make sense of, a situation
- providing feedback to a colleague when they appear to show signs of stress and might benefit from seeking other resources such as counselling or supervision.

However, there are limitations to informal workplace support. Colleagues may be stressed themselves and unable to offer time to listen or show that they care. In addition, they may have been part of the experience that the person is talking about and may impose their own interpretations about the situation.

Structured support in the workplace

Formalised, structured resources in the workplace include:

- support groups
- clinical supervision
- people holding a role that provides mentors/preceptors/educators
- identified resource professionals such as a bereavement coordinator or chaplain
- employer-assisted programme with a counsellor.

In many workplaces, support is provided in some form. Where resources exist, these may be shaped by particular beliefs of managers or the organisation about coping and support. Recently, a midwife in a busy maternity unit explained that all staff had to attend regular support meetings to discuss their feelings about experiences when babies had died. If we think back to Walter's popular guidelines on grief (see p. 36), this appears to reflect a view that everyone must express grief publicly.

As a strategy, it promotes support organisationally; however, at an individual level it might even produce stress for someone who does not wish to focus on loss on that particular day.

Clinical support groups

Just as some bereaved parents find attending mutual help groups useful, some health professionals find it reassuring to know that other colleagues have similar fears and feelings in their practice. The purpose of a clinical support group can vary. It may provide opportunities for reflection, sharing ideas or developing strategies for use in future situations. When establishing a group, there are various points to consider, which can be found in Appendix 13.

We work with colleagues who find such support useful. In some circumstances, groups seek to offer a form of peer supervision. Clinical supervision, whether adapted to a group or with an individual supervisor, may assist to '*identify solutions to problems, improve practice and increase understanding of professional issues*' (United Kingdom Central Council for Nursing, Midwifery and Health Visiting 1996, p. 1). It can be a valuable resource to assist nurses and midwives to cope with stress and loss.

Supervision

Recent studies have found that many health visitors accessed peer support but also wanted advice, support and encouragement from someone trained in bereavement care (Dent et al 1996, Dent 2000).

> *I would have liked debriefing, closer monitoring of visiting pattern and encouragement in clinical supervision from someone knowledgeable and trained.*

> *Although I feel that I am able to support this family, I feel quite isolated in having to carry the 'baggage' that comes with it. Supervision or someone with whom to off-load, would have been very useful.*

We hear similar comments from colleagues attending workshops; supervision is valued and desired. Some have access to supervision as part of their employment; a few fund the costs themselves and many do not have access to this resource. In a recent publication, *Supporting nurses and midwives through lifelong learning*, the Nursing and Midwifery Council (2002) emphasised the importance of clinical supervision for nurses and hoped that such information would be useful to midwives who have their own statutory system of supervision. The Nursing and Midwifery Council document noted that:

- all practitioners should have access to supervision
- supervision should be developed to suit local circumstances
- supervision is an important part of clinical governance to provide quality care.

This has important implications for the practice of nurses and midwives. It means the professional regulatory organisation has stated an expectation for practice in the UK. The question now, is how this resource is provided and funded.

What does supervision offer as a resource? It can provide focused listening time, have an agreement about maintaining confidentiality of information and offer ways to enable people to use their personal resources to explore practice. But does it make a difference? As with bereavement intervention, there are varying models of supervision, outcomes and participants. This hampers conclusions and available information is not necessarily focused on supervision of practitioners providing bereavement care. For example, Carson, Butterworth and Booth (1997, p. 49) evaluated supervision with nurses and noted that the results were '*far from convincing*'. Most importantly, it appears that supervision may work in different ways for different people. Teasdale, Brocklehurst and Thom (2001) found that the supervision helped participants to cope at work, with the greatest difference shown amongst junior nurses. There are varying models for supervision (see Sloan & Watson 2002) and issues involved in the provision of supervision (see Jones 2001). Clearly, the next few years will provide more information about supervision and the ways in which it can be made available to all practitioners.

Questions that a nurse or midwife might consider when approaching a supervisor include:

- what preparation has the supervisor had?
- is the supervisor from within the same profession or work area?
- what is the model or theoretical perspective that underpins the supervision sessions?
- what expectations does the supervisor have of the supervisee and vice versa?
- is supervision open-ended or for time-limited periods?
- are additional supervision sessions available if required by the supervisee because of particular events occurring in practice?
- is supervision available to all staff?

Other sources of workplace support

In some organisations, specifically designated staff offer support to staff members as part of their employment role. This may involve personnel such as a maternity bereavement counsellor, clinical nurse specialist, social worker or chaplain. The success of such a resource may depend on factors including clarifying the purpose of support, defining arrangements to access such support and whether the resource person is perceived as 'safe', without the potential to compromise confidentiality, performance reviews or other working relationships. Some organisations offer funded counselling sessions for employees via employer assisted programmes (EAP). In most circumstances, employees can self-refer and select a counsellor from a specified list, which is followed by attendance at a finite series of sessions to talk about particular issues related to work or home. It can provide a short-term resource, providing a different role to that of clinical supervision.

CULTURAL RESOURCES IN THE WORKPLACE

Working with bereaved families can be one source of challenge and stress within practice. This can affect physical and mental health, which, in turn, may affect work performance, rates of sick leave and even retention of staff. As we have discussed, our perspective is that the ways in which individual health professionals cope with the cost of caring is shaped by personal and social resources. These, in turn, are influenced by beliefs and values from society, government, policy, media and professional organisations. Hence the workplace culture is an important context to coping with stress and loss. Papadatou (2000, p. 72) identified that there may be implicit or explicit rules about expected professional behaviour in the workplace: for example, *'the grief of health professionals must never be so intense as to impair clinical judgement or lead to an emotional breakdown'*. Such rules have the potential to assist or hinder health professionals' grief.

Nurses and midwives might consider whether the organisational culture of their workplace values the cost of care provided by health professionals. Does it have a *'basic aim'* to value and support families and health professionals (Thomas 1999, p. 19). Are there opportunities for:

- education?
- clinical supervision?
- performance review to identify areas for professional development?

As Thomas (1999) noted, valuing families and health professionals requires administration and resources in the workplace setting. Organisational provision of resources such as time to attend supervision or meetings may require a shift in priorities and funding. It is worth considering whether the costs of a workplace culture that values support may be balanced by potential benefits. From the perspective of Capewell and Beattie (1996), support for health professionals has three main aims and it can potentially offer benefits to ensure that:

- bereaved families receive a 'good' service and are protected from a health professional who is unfit emotionally, physically or professionally
- the detrimental effects of work stress on the health of professionals are minimised
- the organisational costs associated with absenteeism and difficulties with retention are reduced.

Health care organisations are made up of individuals, who provide the care to people and their families. As Capewell and Beattie (1996) suggested, the whole is like a Russian doll, where each doll is held and supported at the base by the larger doll, yet each doll has its own space and is a doll in its own right. Hence, as individuals we can care for ourselves, but for maximum benefit we need support in the workplace. The notion of individuals living within contexts is central to this book and we used a similar image to conclude Chapter 2.

Nurses and midwives might consider the ways in which they can contribute to making the organisational culture a caring culture: one that facilitates individual health professionals to cope with stress and loss and be able to continue providing care for bereaved families. As individuals we are not passive; we engage with the resources from social and cultural contexts. We all have the potential to challenge, and possibly change, the values, beliefs and practices in these contexts. One midwife explained the change she initiated in the area where she worked. It offered thoughtful care to bereaved families and also meant that both she and her colleagues were not (di)stressed by having inappropriate equipment.

> *I realised that I was really uncomfortable about not having a suitable 'cot' for very small babies born before 20 weeks. The unit had a small Moses Basket and normal cots, but both were too big for such wee babies. I went out and found a tiny basket and lined it. We now use it for tiny babies and it looks good for taking photographs.*

There are almost certainly strategies that each one of us can think of that we would like to use, initiate or develop for ourselves and our organisation.

SUMMARY

Finally, this text has gone full circle. We started with the family in Chapter 1, where we were reminded that health professionals are members of families too. Our experiences as family members shape who we are and how we provide care. For many of us, our families offer support during times of change and stress at work. We are ending the book with a focus on health professionals and the stressors that may be encountered in the workplace. Equally, many bereaved family members are employed, and they grapple with their bereavement while continuing to be an employee within the workplace. Consequently, this discussion about the workplace can offer a further understanding of contexts that support or constrain the grief of family members.

In conclusion, we believe that for many health professionals the privilege of witnessing grief, caring for others and then integrating these experiences into one's own life can be life-changing. The challenge for individuals is to make meaning of such changes (Montgomery 1993, p. 129):

> *Because caring is always a conscious choice, it is an act of self-actualisation, rather than of self-sacrifice. The reward is the release that comes from losing oneself to the power of something beyond the limits of one's own ego consciousness and the joy of experiencing oneself as part of a greater force...While the task of care-giving can be regulated and controlled, this intangible surrender of caring is beyond control by any authority and therefore is an ultimate expression of freedom and autonomy.*

SUMMARY POINTS

The summary offers an acronym of the main points of this chapter. It is based on REFLECTION, which we see as an important part of dealing with stress and loss (Box 9.1).

Box 9.1

R ecognise your own needs

E xercise body and mind regularly

F ind a trusted colleague to tell your 'story'

L earn relaxation techniques

E at a balanced diet

C ultivate a sense of humour

T ake plenty of water and extra vitamins if necessary

I ndulge yourself every so often

O rganise support for yourself if necessary

N eglect yourself at your peril and that of bereaved families.

This page may be photocopied. We would appreciate acknowledgement to Dent & Stewart (2003) *Sudden death in childhood: support for the bereaved family*. Elsevier Science, Edinburgh

REFERENCES

Capewell E, Beattie L 1996 Staff care and support. In: Lindsey B, Elsegood J (eds) Working with children in grief and loss. Baillière Tindall, London p 162–187

Carson J, Butterworth T, Booth K 1997 Clinical supervision, stress management and social support. In: Butterworth T, Faugier J, Burnard P (eds) Clinical supervision and mentorship in nursing. Stanley Thorne, Cheltenham, UK, p 49–65

Dent A 2000 Support for families whose child dies suddenly from accident or illness. PhD thesis, School of Policy Studies, University of Bristol, UK

Dent A, Condon L, Fleming P et al 1996 A study of bereavement care after sudden and unexpected death. Archives of Disease in Childhood 74: 522–526

Figley CR (ed) 1995 Compassion fatigue: coping with secondary traumatic stress disorder in those who treat the traumatized. Brunner/Mazel, New York

Fontana D 1989 Managing stress. British Psychological Society/Routledge, Leicester, UK

Freudenberger HJ 1974 Staff burnout. Journal of Social Issues 30: 159–165

Jones A 2001 Possible influences on clinical supervision. Nursing Standard 16: 38–42

Montgomery C 1993 Healing through communication. Sage, London

Nursing and Midwifery Council 2002 Code of Professional Conduct. UKCC, London. Available online: http: //www.nmc-uk.org, accessed 1 Feb 2003

Papadatou D 2000 A proposed model of health professionals' grieving process. OMEGA, Journal of Death and Dying 41: 59–77

Riches G, Dawson P 2000 An intimate loneliness: supporting bereaved parents and siblings. Open University Press, Buckingham, UK

Sloan G, Watson H 2002 Clinical supervision models for nursing: structure, research and limitations. Nursing Standard 17: 41–46

Stroebe M, Schut H 1999 The dual process model of coping with bereavement: rationale and description. Death Studies 23: 197–224

Stroebe M, Schut H 2001 Meaning making in the dual process of coping with bereavement. In: Neimeyer R (ed) Meaning reconstruction and the experience of loss. American Psychological Association, Washington, DC, p 55–75

Taylor B 2000 Reflective practice. Allen & Unwin, St Leonards, Australia

Teasdale K, Brocklehurst N, Thom N 2001 Clinical supervision and support for nurses: an evaluation study. Journal of Advanced Nursing 33: 216–224

Thomas J 1999 A baby's death – helping parents make difficult choices. The Practising Midwife 2: 16–19

Tschudin V 1987 Counselling skills for nurses, 2nd edn. Baillière Tindall, London

United Kingdom Central Council (UKCC) 1996 Position statement on clinical supervision for nursing and health visiting. UKCC, London. Available online: http//www.nmc-org.uk, accessed 1 Feb 2003

Wagner J T, Higdon T 1996 Spiritual issues and bioethics in the intensive care unit: the role of chaplain. Critical Care Clinics 12: 15–27

Walter T 1999 On bereavement: the culture of grief. Open University Press, Buckingham, UK

Williams G, Lowe L 2000 Reflection: possible strategies to improve its use by qualified staff. British Journal of Nursing 10: 1482–1488

USEFUL SOURCES FOR NURSES AND MIDWIVES

Bailey R, Clarke M 1989 Stress and coping in nursing Chapman & Hall, London

Burnard P 1997 Know yourself! Self awareness activities for nurses and other health professionals. Whurr, London

Montgomery C 1993 Healing through communication Sage, Newbury Park, UK

Appendices

1 National organisations to help bereaved parents

Organisations offer a range of services such as written information leaflets to give to families, helplines, befrienders and group meetings. Brief details describe each organisation. Further information can be obtained by contacting the organisation directly. Details are for the UK unless otherwise stated. Every effort has been made for the information to be accurate at the time of going to press.

Alder Centre
Royal Liverpool Children's NHS Trust
Alder Hey
Eaton Rd, Liverpool L12 2AP
Tel: 0151 252 9759
This organisation provides support, information and training for all those affected by the death of a child.

ARC (Antenatal results and choices, formerly known as SATFA)
73–75 Charlotte St
London SW1P 1LB
Tel: 0207 6310285
Website: www.arc-uk.org
The organisation offers support to parents for fetal abnormality and termination.

Belt Up School Kids (bus/coach/minibus crashes)
18 Windsor Rd, Newcastle
Gwent NP19 8NS
Tel: 01633 274944
This organisation offers support to families whose children have been involved in road crashes.

Bliss
68 South Lambeth Rd, London SE1 7TP
Tel: 0870 7700337
Helpline Tel: 0500 618140 (9.30 a.m. to 5.30 p.m. Mondays to Fridays)
Website: www.bliss.org.uk
This organisation offers support to families whose children are in special care baby units.

Brake Care
PO Box 548
Huddersfield HD1 2XZ
Tel: 01484 559983
Email: brakecare@brake.org.uk
This organisation has published a booklet 'Coping with grief – when someone you love is killed on the road'.

British Association of Counselling
1 Regent Place
Rugby CV21 2PJ
Information line: 01788 578328
Email: bac@bac.co.uk
Website: www.bacp.co.uk
The association provides a list of approved counsellors in each area. Each counsellor will operate a sliding scale of charges.

Campaign Against Drinking and Driving
39 Heaton Rd
Newcastle NE6 1SB
Tel: 0191 265 7147
This is a pressure group to abolish drinking and driving.

Child Bereavement Trust
Aston House
High St
West Wycombe
High Wycombe, Bucks HP14 3AG
General enquiries: 01494 446648
Information and support line: 0845 3571000
Email: enquiries@childbereavement.org.uk
Website: www.childbereavement.org.uk
The trust offers bereaved parents and children: leaflets, videos, books, activity packs for children and memory boxes.

Child Death Help-line
Great Ormond St Hospital, London
And Alder Hey Hospital, Liverpool
Freephone (both): 0800 282 9869639 (7 p.m. to 10 p.m. every evening and 10 a.m. to 1 p.m. Monday, Wednesday and Friday)
Website: www.ich.ucl.ac.uk
The helpline offers confidential emotional support from trained bereaved parents to anyone affected by the death of a child, from any cause.

The Compassionate Friends
53 North St
Bristol BS3 1EN
Tel: 0117 953 9639
Website: www.tcf.org.uk
It has a network of support groups for bereaved parents throughout the UK run by bereaved parents and offers a wide range of leaflets on bereavement.

The Compassionate Friends Australia
Victoria contact:
www.compassionatefriendsvictoria.org.au
New South Wales contact:
www.thecompassionatefriends.org.au

Cruse Bereavement Care
Cruse House
126 Sheen Rd
Richmond
Surrey TW9 1UR

Tel: 0208 9399530
Website: www.crusebereavementcare.org.uk
This organisation offers support to anyone who has been bereaved. There is a network of support groups throughout the UK and it offers a wide range of leaflets on bereavement. The Cruse website has a page 'specially for schools' and is also running a project called the Youth Involvement Project, which can be found on the website: www.rd4.org.uk.

Ectopic Pregnancy Trust
Maternity Unit
Hillingdon Hospital
Pield Health Rd
Uxbridge UB8 3NN
Helpline: 01895 238 025
Website: www.ectopic.org.uk
This organisation provides support and information.

Foundation for the Study of Infant Deaths (FSID)
Artillery House
11–19 Artillery Row
London SW1P 1RT
Tel: 0870 7870885
Email: support@sids.org.uk
Helpline 0870 7870554 (9 a.m. to 11 p.m. Mondays to Fridays; 6 p.m. to 11 p.m. Saturday and Sunday)
Website: www.sids.org.uk
This organisation offers a helpline for parents and professionals and has a wide network of befrienders for families throughout the UK. Free phone cards are available to bereaved families. It has a wide range of leaflets.

Meningitis Research Foundation
Midland Way
Thornbury
Bristol BS35 2BS
24 hour helpline: 080 88003344
Website: www.meningitis.org
This organisation offers help and support to parents whose child has died from meningitis.

Miscarriage Association
c/o Clayton Hospital
Northgate
Wakefield

West Yorkshire WF1 3JS
Tel: 01924 200799
Website: www.the-ma.org.uk
*This organisation runs a national helpline and
has a network of support groups and information
leaflets.*

Miscarriage Association New Zealand

www.miscarriage.org.nz
*Through the country there are local group meetings,
information is available to support families.*

National Meningitis Trust

Fern House
Bath Rd
Stroud GL5 3TJ
General enquiries: 01453 768000
Helpline: 0345 7538118
*This organisation offers support to families when
a child has died from meningitis.*

Retained Organs Commission

PO Box 32794, London SE1 6WA
Helpline: 0800 0920203
Email: Retained-Organs-Commission@doh.
gsi.gov.uk

RoadPeace

PO Box 2579, London NW10 3PW
Tel: 0208 964 1021
*The organisation is for all road traffic victims and
their families.*

Samaritans

The Upper Mill
Kingston Rd
Ewell
Surrey KT17 2AF
General office (enquiries only): 0208 3948301
Helpline for bereavement support: 08457 909090
Email: jo@samaritans.org
Website: www.samaritans.org.uk
*The helpline, run by trained volunteers, is open
24 hours a day and is available to anyone in need.*

SAMM (Support after Murder and Manslaughter)

Cranmer House
39 Buxton Road
London SW9 6 DZ
Tel: 020 7735 3838
Website: www.samm.org.uk
*This organisation offers support to families and has
assisted the Home Office in developing a Homicide
Information Pack. It is also involved in education,
public awareness and supporting research.*

SANDS (Stillbirth and Neonatal Death Society)

28 Portland Place
London WIN 4DE
Tel: 0270 4365881
Website: www.uk-sands.org
*This organisation provides support to parents who have
lost a baby during late pregnancy or around birth.
There is a network of support groups throughout UK
and has a wide range of leaflets.*

SANDS Australia National Council

Suite 208, 901 White Horse Rd
Boxhill Victoria 3128
Australia
Website: www.sands.org.au
*This organisation offers group meetings, education,
conference, newsletter for families after stillbirth,
miscarriage and neonatal death.*

SANDS New Zealand

SANDS Auckland
PO Box 90034
Auckland Mail Centre
Auckland
Tel: 09 4461144
*This organisation has local groups throughout the
country and offers a newsletter.*

Scottish Cot Death Trust

Royal Hospital
Yorkhill
Glasgow G3 8SJ
Tel: 0141 3573946

Website: www.gla.ac.uk.departments/
childhealth.SCDT
This organisation raises money to initiate and fund research into the causes and prevention of cot death. It offers support to bereaved families and a range of information leaflets.

SIDS Australia
www.sidsaustralia.org.nz
Throughout Australia; there are local groups, resources, education and research.

SIDS International
www.sidsinternational.minerva.com.au
Provides information on research, conferences and links to SIDS support organisations in different countries.

Survivors of Bereavement by Suicide (SOBS)
Centre 88
Saner St
Hull HU3 2TR
Tel: 01482 210287
Website: www.uk-sobs.org.uk
This organisation offers support to those who have experienced suicide and has an informative leaflet for survivors.

The Sudden Infant Death Charitable Trust (New Zealand)
Tel: 0800 743754
This organisation offers nationwide support, counselling and infant health information.

TAMBA (Twins and Multiple Births Association)
Harnott House
309 Chester Rd
Little Sutton
Ellesmere Port
CH66 1QQ
Tel: 0870 7703304
Website: www.tamba.org.uk
This organisation offers a network of support throughout the UK. It also provides information and publications.

The Trauma After-Care Trust (TACT)
Buttfields
The Farthings
Withington
Glos GL54 4DF
Tel: 01242 890306
The trust holds a list of carers in most areas of UK where severe trauma has occurred.

Victim Support
PO Box 1143
London SW9 6ZH
Tel: 0845 3030900
Website: www.victimsupport.com (redirects to Scotland, England and Wales, Republic of Ireland sites)
This organisation offers a network of experienced volunteers throughout most parts of the UK to help those bereaved as a result of crime.

Winston's Wish
The Clara Burgess Centre
Gloucestershire Royal Hospital
Great Western Rd
Gloucester GL1 3NN
Family Line: 0845 2030405
General enquiries: 01452 394377
Email: info@winstonswish.org.uk
Website: www.winstonswish.org.uk
This organisation provides support for bereaved children up to 18 years and their parents or carers. All services are free to families in Gloucestershire. For people living outside the county, the organisation can be contacted for further details.

Woodland Trust
Autumn Park
Dysart Rd
Grantham
Lincs NG31 6LL
Tel: 0147 6581111
The trust offers to plant trees as a memorial.

National organisations for bereaved children

Organisations offer a range of services such as written information leaflets to give to families and helplines. Brief details describe each organisation, further information can be obtained by contacting the organisation directly. Every effort has been made for the information to be accurate at the time of going to press.

Candle Project
St Christopher's Hospice
51–59 Lawrie Park Rd
London SE26 6DZ
Tel: 020 87684500
Website: www.stchristophers.org.uk
This organisation offers one to one and group counselling for children, young people and families in Southeast London and has resources for parents and professionals.

Childhood Bereavement Network
Huntingdon House, 278–290 Huntingdon St
Nottingham NG1 3LY
Tel: 0115 9118070
Email: cbn@ncb.org.uk
This is an umbrella organisation to link together individuals and agencies who are working with bereaved children and their families. It offers information and a list of services involved with supporting bereaved children throughout UK.

Child Bereavement Trust
Aston House
High St
West Wycombe

High Wycombe
Bucks HP14 3AG
General enquiries: 01494 446648
Information and support line: 0845 3571000
Email: enquiries@childbereavement.org.uk
Website: www.childbereavement.org.uk
The trust offers leaflets, videos, books, activity packs for children and memory boxes for bereaved parents and children.

Childline
Studd St, London N1 0QW
Tel: 0207 2391000
For Children: Freepost, 111 London N1 0BR
Tel: 0800 1111 (24 hour helpline)
Website: www.childline.org.uk
This organisation offers help and support to any child or young person including bereaved children.

Cruse Bereavement Care
Cruse House
126 Sheen Rd
Richmond
Surrey TW9 1UR
Tel: 0208 9399530
Website: www.crusebereavementcare.org.uk
Young people can telephone free on 0808 081677
(Wednesdays 4 p.m. to 7 p.m. or leave a message at any time)
This organisation offers free support to anyone who has been bereaved. There is a network of support groups throughout the UK and it has a wide range of leaflets on bereavement. The Cruse website has a page

'specially for schools' and is also running a project called the Youth Involvement Project, which can be found on www.rd4.org.uk.

Daisy's Dream

PO Box 4738
Twyford, Reading
Berkshire RG10 9GT
Tel: 0118 9342604
Email: info@daisysdream.org.uk
This organisation offers support and advice nationally by telephone.

Notre Dame Centre

20 Athole Gardens
Glasgow G12 9BA
Tel: 0141 3392366
Email: notredamecentre@tesco.net
This organisation provides initial consultation to families by telephone. A consultancy service is also available. Services can be tailormade and delivered on a Scotland-wide basis. They run 'Seasons for growth', which is a loss and grief peer-support programme for children from 6 to 18 years. They also run the Raft Project, which is a specialised trauma service for children who are experiencing post-traumatic stress symptoms.

Tree Tops

Corrymeela House, 8 Upper Crescent
Belfast BT7 1NT
Tel: 028 90508080
Email: info@bereavedchild.org
Website: www.bereavedchild.org
This organisation offers a support programme for small groups of children between the ages of 8 and 12 years to meet other bereaved children to share their experiences. Parents are asked to come too and meet separately. They also offer a magazine, which includes stories, poems, drawings and letters from bereaved children.

Winston's Wish

The Clara Burgess Centre
Gloucestershire Royal Hospital
Great Western Rd
Gloucester GL1 3NN
Tel: 0845 2030405
Email: info@winstonswish.org.uk
Website: www.winstonswish.org.uk
This organisation provides support for bereaved children up to 18 years and their parents or carers. All services are free to families in Gloucestershire. For people living outside the county, the organisation can be contacted for further details.

3 Websites on bereavement

Websites are available 24 hours per day and offer information, links to other sites and chatrooms. Further sites are listed with organisations in Appendices 1 and 2.

Alliance of Grandparents A Support in Tragedy
www.agast.org
Offers resources, support and information for all grandparents who have had a grandchild die.

Bereaved Parents USA
www.bereavedparents.usa.org
Monthly meetings, newsletters open to parents, siblings and grandparents.

Centering Corporation
www.centering.org
Has extensive range of books for sale, based in US; also offers links to other grief sites.

Grief Recovery Online for all Bereaved
http://www.groww.com
Provides chat rooms, information and links to other sites.

Internet support group
www.griefnet.org

Mothers Against Drink Driving
www.madd.org
Based in US it provides resources, information and statistics.

Parents of Murdered Children
www.pomc.com
Offers online support, group meetings, education and legal information.

Resources for bereaved children and their parents

Where possible brief details describe each item; further information can be obtained by contacting the provider directly. Every effort has been made for the information to be accurate at the time of going to press.

Games for bereaved children
All about me
Produced by Peta Hemmings
Available from Barnardos, Tel: 0208 5508822
A useful resource for adults working with primary school children.

The grief game
Y Searle & I Streng, Published by Jessica Kingsley, London.

Videos
Someone died: it happened to me
Price £15.50
Available from Child Bereavement Trust
Tel: 01494 446648
For bereaved children and teenagers. Girls and boys from 7 to 18 years discuss their feelings. Parents talk too.

When a child grieves
Price £25.00, excl p&p
Available from Child Bereavement Trust
Tel: 01494 446648

For parents, carers and professionals. It invites carers to listen to the experience of bereaved children and gives advice on how to respond to the needs of families. It also shows how to introduce death in the classroom.

That morning I went to school
Price £16.50, incl p&p
Available from Northamptonshire Social Services
Tel: 01604 545131
Bereaved children relate their experiences.

A Death in the Lives of...
Price £12.50
Available from Child Bereavement Network
Tel: 0115 9118070
A group of children aged 13–16 years talk about support that helped them to cope with bereavement. It raises awareness of children's needs and ways that can provide information and support.

Grief in the family
Price £10 for hire
Available from Leeds Animation Workshop
Tel: 0113 2484997
This animated video looks at ways children and young people respond to grief and what adults can do to help them. It gives an insight into the process of grieving, its physical and emotional effects and the special needs of children.

Books for bereaved parents and grandparents

Every effort has been made for details to be accurate at the time of going to press. Many books overlap the broad categories below and relate to death of a baby and a child. Many of the organisations listed below and in Appendices 1 and 2 (also funeral directors) provide pamphlets for bereaved parents, siblings, grandparents and friends.

Availability of texts and resources

In all countries, bookshops are able to order books.

Amazon Books

www.amazon.com
Older editions of books may be able to be sourced from Amazon.

Centering Corporation

1531 North Saddle Creek Rd.
Omaha NE 68104 USA
www.centering.org
Sells a wide range of texts and resources for all ages.

Thanatos Books

PO Box 134, Manchester M8 4DJ
Tel: 0161 7401335
www.thanatosbooks.seekbooks.co.uk
A bookshop that specialises in such texts in the UK

General grief

Caplan S, Lang G 1995 Grief's courageous journey. New Harbinger, Oakland, CA

Heaney P 2002 Coming to grief. Longacre Press, Dunedin, NZ

The death of a child

Cooper A, Harpin V 1991 This is our child: how parents experience the medical world. Oxford University Press, Oxford

Farrant A 1998 Sibling bereavement. Cassell, London

Finkbeiner AK 1996 After the death of a child: living with loss through the years. Johns Hopkins University Press, Baltimore, MD

Fox L 2000 I have no intention of saying goodbye: parents share their stories of hope and healing after a child's death. Universe

Gatenby B 1998 For the rest of our lives after the death of a child. Reed Books, Auckland, NZ

Hindmarch C 2000 On the death of a child, 2nd edn. Radcliffe Medical Press, Oxford

Jurgensen G 1999 The disappearance. Harper Collins, London (*The death of author's daughters aged 4 and 7 in a road traffic accident*)

McCraken A, Semel M (eds) 1998 A broken heart still beats: after your child dies. Hazelden, Center City, MN

Madill B 2001 One step at a time. Floris Books, Edinburgh (*Author's 3-year-old daughter died in swimming pool accident*)

Rosenblatt PC 2000 Help your marriage survive the death of a child. Temple University Press, Philadelphia, PA

Ruskin D 2002 A candle for Lisa. Pennine Pens, Pennine, PA (*Heart defect in premature baby: organs retained by pathology department*)

Sarnoff Schiff H 1977 The bereaved parent. Souvenir Press, London

Smith S 1999 When you walk through a storm. Mainstream, Edinburgh (*An account of mother's reaction to son's death at the Hillsborough Stadium disaster in 1989*)

Talbot K 2002 What forever means after the death of a child. Brunner-Routledge, New York

Winston's Wish 2002 Beyond the rough rock: supporting a child who has been bereaved through suicide. Available from Winston's Wish (see Organisations)

Death of a baby

Boyle MF 1997 Mothers bereaved by stillbirth, neonatal death or sudden infant death syndrome. Ashgate, Aldershot, UK

Kohner N, Henley A 2001 When a baby dies, 2nd edn. Routledge, London

Nicol M 1997 Loss of a baby. Death of a dream. Harper Collins, Sydney

Sudden infant death syndrome (SIDS)

Deveson-Lord J 1987 When a baby suddenly dies. Hill of Content, Melbourne

Horchler J, Rice Morris R 1997 The SIDS survival guide. SIDS Educational Services, Hyattsville MD

Miscarriage

Faldet R, Fitton K (eds) 1997 Our stories of miscarriage. Fairview Press, Minneapolis

Hey V, Itzin C, Saunders L, Speakman M (eds) 1996 Hidden loss. The Women's Press, London (*Includes ectopic pregnancy*)

Kluger-Bell K 2000 Unspeakable losses. Harper Collins, Sydney

Kohner N, Henley A 2001 When a baby dies, 2nd edn. Routledge, London

Moulder C 2001 Miscarriage: women's experiences and needs, 3rd edn. Routledge, London

Oakley A, McPherson A, Roberts H 1984 Miscarriage. Penguin, London

Regan L 2001 Miscarriage, what every woman wants to know, 2nd edn. Orion, London

Saunders L 1996 Hidden loss: miscarriage and ectopic pregnancy. The Women's Press, London

Late miscarriage, stillbirth and neonatal death

Hill S 1989 Family. Penguin, London

Kohner N, Henley A 2001 When a baby dies, 2nd edn. Routledge, London

Memory resources

Ferguson D 1989 Little footprints; a special baby's memory book. Centering Corporation, Omaha NE (*Contains structured headings and questions against which information about birth and death of a baby can be written with room for journal entries, comments about the funeral, anniversary. There are short verses and illustrative images*)

Booklets/books specifically written for grandparents

Cerza Kolf J 1995 Grandma's tears. Baker Books, Grand Rapids, MI

Gerner M 1990 For bereaved grandparents. Centering Corporation, Omaha, NE

Leininger L, Ilse S 1985 Grieving grandparents. Pregnancy and Infant Loss Center, Wayzata, MN

6 Books for bereaved children and young people

Availability of texts and resources is given in Appendix 5.

General

Amos J 1997 Separations: death. Cherrytree, Slough, UK

Bryant-Mole K 1998 What do we think about death? Hodder & Stoughton, London

Cathcart F 1996 Understanding death and dying: your feelings. British Institute of Learning Disabilities, London www.bild.org.uk

Connolly M 1997 It isn't easy. Oxford University Press, Oxford

Grollman EA 1991 Talking about death: a dialogue between parent and child, 3rd edn. Beacon, Oklahoma City, OK

Grollman EA 1993 Straight talk about death for teenagers. Beacon, Oklahoma City, OK

Grollman EA 1996 Living when a young friend commits suicide. Beacon, Oklahoma City, OK

Heegaard M 1988 When someone very special dies. Woodland Press, Minneapolis, MN

Johnson J 1997 How do I feel about: my step-family. Franklin Watts, London

For younger children

Brown LK 1996 When dinosaurs die: a guide to understanding death. Time Warner

Buscaglia L 1983 The fall of Freddie the leaf. Holt, Rinehart & Winston, New York

Cohn J 1987 I had a friend named Peter: talking to children about the death of a friend. William Morrow, New York (*Betsy's friend is killed by a car*)

Harper A 1994 Remembering Michael. SANDS, London (see organisations) (*A baby brother dies at birth*)

Heegaard M 1991 When someone very special dies. Woodland Press, Minnesota, MN (*Helping children to illustrate their own story and feelings*)

Varley S 1985 Badger's parting gifts. Hodder & Stoughton, London (*Remembering a loved friend*)

Williams M 1975 The velveteen rabbit. Camelot Books, Bristol (*A book to be read with parents, to reassure children of their love*)

Books for learning disabled children

Cathcart F 1994 Understanding death and dying. British Institute of Learning Disability, Kidderminster (Tel: 0156 272 3010 or www.bild.org.uk)

Morris L 1996 Remembering my brother. A&C Black, London

Helping parents support their surviving children

S upply information about the death as soon as possible

U nderstand that they grieve in their own way

P rovide careful and sensitive listening if at all possible

P reserve routine activities and boundaries

O ffer choices after explanations (e.g. seeing the body, going to the funeral)

R eassure that they are not to blame

T alk through their fears and anxieties

I nvolve and include whenever possible without giving too many responsibilities

N urture and share moments together; parents can provide a grieving model (e.g. crying together is OK)

G ive opportunities to remember the dead person (memory box, photos, scrap book)

This page may be photocopied. It is presented here in adapted form and is not copyrighted. We would appreciate acknowledgement to Dent & Stewart (2003) *Sudden death in childhood: support for the bereaved family*. Elsevier Science, Edinburgh

Resources for health professionals working with children and families

Useful reading

Bayliss, J 1996 Understanding loss and grief. National Extension College, Cambridge
The Michael Young Centre, Purbeck Rd, Cambridge
Website: www.nec.ac.uk
This is a training pack, including exercises which are able to be photocopied.

Cruse: Supporting bereaved children and families
Cruse House, 126 Sheen Rd, Richmond,
Surrey TW9 1UR
This is a training manual available from the Cruse organisation (see Appendix 1).

Kohner N, Leftwich A 1995 A pregnancy loss and the death of a baby. National Extension College, Cambridge
The Michael Young Centre, Purbeck Rd, Cambridge
Website: www.nec.ac.uk
This includes SANDS updated guidelines for professionals.

Lindsey B, Elsegood J (eds) 1996 Working with children in loss and grief. Baillière-Tindall, London
Offers professionals working with children opportunities to increase their awareness of children's grief, ways to help children and an understanding of when to seek expert help.

Machin L 1993 Working with young people in loss situations. Pavilion Press, Brighton
8 St Georges Place, Brighton B21 4ZZ

Tel: 01273 623222
This offers practical material, including picture triggers and work-sheets for working with children.

Morgan J 2001 Social support: a reflection of humanity. Baywood, Amityville, NY
Various chapters about the role of social support including working with bereaved children and schools, and following suicide. Differentiates support from other forms of intervention such as therapy.

Smith S, Pennells M (eds) 1995 Interventions with bereaved children. Jessica Kinglsey, London
Covers different approaches in working with bereaved children. Play therapy, group, individual and family work, work with adolescents are all discussed.

Ward B 1995 Good grief: exploring feelings, loss and death, 2nd edn. Jessica Kinglsey, London
Vol 1 is for under 11s; Vol 2 for over 11s and adults.

Videos for professionals
Childhood grief
£16.50 incl p&p
Available from Gill Schofield, Tel: 01604 545131
Endeavours to assist social workers teachers and other professionals to understand more fully the complexities of children's grief.

Life Goes On

£17.62

Available from St Margaret's Hospice Taunton

Tel: 01823 345907

Four teenage girls talk about their personal experience of bereavement with reference to friends, school and family members.

A Portrait of Family Grief

£60 incl p&p

Available from Acorns Children's Hospice

Tel: 0121 2484800

Giving Sorrow Words

Available from Video Inset, PO Box 197

Cardiff CF5 2WF

Useful for staff training or individual teachers. Deals with breaking the news of a death and helping children to return to school after bereavement.

Websites/organisations

Association for Death and Counselling

www.adec.org

Offers newsletter, conferences, publications, education that may be of use to health professionals.

Bereavement Research Forum

Christina Mason (Secretary)

St Joseph's Hospice

More St

Hackney

London E8 4SA

UK

Tel: 020 8525 6000

email: emason@srjh.org.uk

The forum is a membership organisation offering three symposia yearly on different aspects of bereavement research. A conference is held biannually. There are opportunities for members to network, to learn about research and to discuss and be supported in their current or intended research.

Centre for Grief Education

McCulloch House, Monash Medical Centre

246 Clayton Rd, Clayton Victoria 3168, Australia

Website: www.grief.org.au

Provides information on projects, bereavement support directory, journal, counselling and education.

Child Bereavement Trust

Aston House, High St, West Wycombe,

High Wycombe, Bucks HP14 3AG

General enquiries: 01494 446648

Information and support line: 0845 3571000

Offers training for health professionals on a wide range of bereavement issues concerning the death of a child.

Growth House

Website: www.growthhouse.org/death.html

Provides chat room, professionals forum, information and links to other sites.

National Association for Loss and Grief (Australia)

Website: www.NALAG-griefaustralia.org

Goal to enable community to recognise loss and change in life. The group promotes resources, education and research.

Winston's Wish

The Clara Burgess Centre, Gloucestershire Royal Hospital, Great Western Rd, Gloucester GL1 3NN

Tel: 0845 2030405

Produces a range of activities for working with bereaved children, and also guidelines for teachers involved in a school-related death.

9 Taking photographs

To maximise the success of taking photographs, decisions include choice of camera, number of photographs taken, photographer and picture composition.

The choice of camera

Plan to use several cameras if possible to ensure that photographs are available even if one camera fails to perform. It may be useful to use two types of camera that have different advantages. A polaroid camera will produce instant photographs, which can be valuable to families who have no other photographs, such as when a baby is stillborn. These photographs do deteriorate over time. However, photographic services can create further prints or images from the original photograph. A digital camera creates images that can be emailed to friends and integrated into documents such as memory cards. Most frequently, cameras with print film are used and the negatives can be used to reproduce multiple sets of photographs.

The number of photographs

Always take **lots** of photographs. Some will come out well; others will not and there are limited opportunities to take photographs before the funeral. It can be worth having films processed separately at different times, since if any mishaps occur during processing there will still be another back-up film.

The photographer

Health professionals, family members and professional photographers (for a fee) can all take the role of photographer. Clearly all have varying skills and familiarity with the equipment. This needs to be considered since there are only limited opportunities to secure successful photographs before the funeral of the child.

The picture composition

It is worth taking a moment to consider how the photograph will appear in the future. Considerations described in setting the scene for families to see their child (p. 141) are relevant here.

Background colour in relation to the child. Bright red skin of a premature baby can contrast unfavourably with green sheets, whereas pale, cyanosed skin does not contrast with white sheets.

Setting of the photograph. Is it a clinical environment? Can it be adapted to have a softer, home-like setting?

Use of clothes. Are there particular clothes that the parents would like the child to wear? Will they then keep these clothes as part of their mementos?

Focus of the picture. Encourage family members to look at the child when the photograph is being taken. Photographs can be taken from different perspectives, with the camera pointed directly at the child and also at an angle. Parents may want a range of photographs such as:

- the child alone
- the child both dressed and naked, if the latter is acceptable to the family
- parts of the child, e.g. a perfect hand or ear
- the child held by/with different members of the family individually and together as a group
- significant health professionals (such as a midwife) with the child/baby.

Use of a flash light. Is it possible to get sufficient light without a flash? A flash can create harsher images.

10 Planning a funeral

At the service, there are many options that families might wish to consider:

- having a family-only or public service
- religious or humanistic perspective
- clergy, celebrant, family member or other person conducting the service
- taking the child to the service in a family car or a hearse
- having an open casket or not
- offering people the chance to put items in the casket (photographs, stories, toys, mementos of significance)
- lining the casket
- selecting particular clothes for the child to wear

- family members carrying the casket in and out of the service
- family members making the casket
- poems and songs or particular significance to the family or child
- music of significance
- photographing, audio or videotaping the service
- symbolic farewell such as releasing balloons or homing pigeons at the end of the service
- having a tribute book for people at the funeral to sign
- asking people to place a flower on top of the casket
- flower arrangements with a particular theme associated with the child.

A bereavement assessment tool

Currently the questions are framed towards parent(s). These can be adapted to suit other family members.

About the death

How were the parents told of the death? Were they present at the death? Did the hospital staff give good care before the death? Were the parents kept fully informed as to what was happening? Were the parents satisfied with the Emergency Services? Were they satisfied with any care given by religious leaders in hospital?

After the death

Were the parents able to stay with their child for as long as they wanted? Were they given an opportunity of holding/washing/dressing their child? Were they given any tokens of remembrance, e.g. photographs, hand and foot prints, lock of hair? Did their other children have the opportunity of seeing the dead child and saying goodbye in an unhurried way?

Postmortem and coroner (if applicable)

How did the parents feel about their contact with the coroner's officer? Were the findings of the postmortem/coroner's investigation explained clearly? Do they have any outstanding questions?

Information and follow-up

Have the parents been given any information by health professionals/others about grief, the cause of death, registering the death, arranging the funeral, mutual help groups? If appropriate, were the parents given a follow-up appointment to see a doctor at the hospital to talk of the death?

The funeral

Was (is) the funeral director/ spiritual leader helpful? If there are other children, did they/will they attend the funeral? How do (did) the parents feel about the funeral?

The media

Has the media caused any problems for the family?

Relationships with members of the close family

Parents
Are the parents able to talk together about the death? Are they finding they have different feelings at different times from each other? Are they able to be close to each other during this time?

Grandparents

Are the grandparents able to talk about the death with the parents? Do they have different attitudes to the death? Are the grandparents able to help support the parents/other children? Do the grandparents need support or information?

Other children

What do the children know about the death? Do the parents have difficulty in talking with them? Are the parents able to share their emotions with their children? Have they involved them in activities/rituals to mark the death of the child?

Support from friends, neighbours and other family members

What support is available from other family members, friends and neighbours? Do the parents feel they have sufficient support? Do friends and others outside the close family avoid them? Do the parents feel isolated and let down by them?

Practical difficulties

Are there any practical problems that are causing difficulty for the parents at the present? What would help the parents?

Schools and community groups (where appropriate)

Do the schools/playgroups of other siblings know about the death? Are the parents able to talk to the other children's teachers/play-leaders about the death? Do other parents at school/playgroup talk with, or avoid, the parents?

Health

Do the parents usually have good health? Has their appetite, sleeping or energy level been affected after the death? Has either of the parents suffered from depression in the past?

Past losses

Has the mother had a miscarriage, termination or stillbirth in the past? If so, are there still painful memories? Have the parents experienced deaths of close family members or friends recently, some time ago, or as a child? Do these deaths still cause pain? Have there been other recent changes in the family such as divorce, redundancy?

Spiritual

Do the parents believe in a God/higher being/spiritual meaning of life? Do they feel angry with God? Do they wonder where their child is now? Would they like to talk to a priest/vicar/spiritual leader/someone else about the death? What meaning has the death for each member of the family?

Do the parents have any particular fears at the present?

Are there any other areas of concern for the parents?

What do parents perceive as the strengths of the family?

What do parents perceive as the needs of the family?

This page may be photocopied.
We would appreciate acknowledgement to Dent & Stewart (2003) *Sudden death in childhood: support for the bereaved family*. Elsevier Science, Edinburgh

The information from the tool can be used to plan care; this might include documentation in a care plan such as the following list. Or it might include assessment and documentation in another form.

Care plan for prioritising stresses and resources in the family

Stresses/resources	Score		
	1	2	3
About the death			
After the death			
Postmortem and coroner			
Information and follow-up			
The funeral			
The media			
Relationships			
Partner			
Surviving children			
Grandparents			
Friends			
Schools			
Teachers			
Other parents			
School friends			
Health			
Support			
Partner			
Family			
Friends			
Past losses			
Spiritual issues			
Practical problems			
Fears of parents			

1 is the highest priority at any one time, 3 the lowest.

This page may be photocopied.
We would appreciate acknowledgement to Dent & Stewart (2003) *Sudden death in childhood: support for the bereaved family.* Elsevier Science, Edinburgh

12 Complexities of grieving

This section provides an overview with references for further reading about complicated grief, post-traumatic stress and suicide.

Complicated grief

As we discussed in earlier chapters, language shapes expectations and understandings. Descriptors of grief have included 'abnormal' or 'pathological'. The more recent use of the term 'complicated' indicates the potential for mourning to become 'uncomplicated' (Rando, 1992, 1993). Rando, a clinical psychologist with extensive clinical experience with bereaved parents, has written about complicated mourning (rather than grief) and we have used this term in this section of the book. She has provided an excellent resource on complicated mourning. This provides detail of working with bereaved people in both complicated and uncomplicated mourning.

So what is complicated grief? It is a judgement based on assessment of another person's experience in relation to expected pattern(s) of grieving. As the discussion in Chapter 2 indicated, *expected* patterns are located within social beliefs and values that change over time. There are tensions in making assessments about others' experiences. We believe it is not generally within the scope of practice of health visitors and midwives working with bereaved families to make a diagnosis of complicated grief. Rather, it is to be aware that some family members may be extremely distressed and may find benefit from another person skilled in working with the bereaved. Rando's work provides a framework to consider when mourning may be complicated or difficult.

From Rando's perspective, complicated mourning is '*some compromise, distortion or failure of one or more of the six R processes*' (1993, p. 149).

These are described in more detail on p. 30. Therefore, complicated mourning is defined in relation to the **reference point** of the six R processes. It is one perspective of grief, as we noted in Chapter 2.

Rando also offered some indicators of complicated mourning. These need to be considered in relation to:

- the R processes: are these compromised or distorted?
- the particular mourner and the loss
- the time since the death.

(From Rando T 1993 *Treatment of complicated mourning*. Research Press, Illinois, pp. 152–153. With permission of T. Rando, copyright holder.)

Clinical indicators of complicated mourning

1. A pattern of vulnerability to, sensitivity toward or overreaction to experiences entailing loss and separation.
2. Psychological and behavioural restlessness, oversensitivity, arousal, overreactivity and perception of being 'geared up', along with the need always to be occupied, as if cessation of movement would permit the surfacing of anxiety-provoking repressed or suppressed material.
3. Unusually high death anxiety focusing on the self or loved ones.

4. Excessive and persistent overidealization of the deceased and/or unrealistically positive recollections of the relationship.

5. Rigid, compulsive, or ritualistic behaviour sufficient to impinge on the mourner's freedom and well-being.

6. Persistent obsessive thoughts and preoccupation with the deceased and elements of the loss.

7. Inability to experience the various emotional reactions to loss typically found in the bereaved and/or uncharacteristically constricted affect.

8. Inability to articulate, to whatever capacity the mourner has, existing feelings and thoughts about the deceased and the loss.

9. Relationships with others marked by fear of intimacy and other indices of avoidance stemming primarily from fear of future loss.

10. A pattern of self-destructive relationships commencing or escalating subsequent to the death, including compulsive caregiving and replacement relationships.

11. The commencement or escalation after the death of self-defeating, self-destructive, or acting-out behaviour, including psychoactive substance dependence or abuse.

12. Chronic experience of numbness, alienation, depersonalisation, or other affects and occurrences that isolate the mourner from her/himself and others.

13. Chronic anger or some variation thereof (e.g. annoyance) or a combination of anger and depression (e.g. irritability, belligerence, intolerance).

Post-traumatic stress

Rando (1996) has also offered a reminder that post-traumatic stress may be part of the experience of some bereaved family members. She defined trauma, using Figley's work, as '*an emotional state of discomfort and stress resulting from memories of an extraordinary catastrophic experience which shattered the survivor's sense of invulnerability to harm*' (Rando 1996, p. 144). Using this definition encompasses some situations where a child has died unexpectedly. Some family members may experience traumatic images of the death, which may result from being present at the death or having limited information about the circumstances of the death (Lord 1996). As Rando (1996) noted, many bereaved family members do not have short-term post-traumatic stress reactions or post-traumatic stress disorder. However, nurses and midwives need to consider this possibility, which might include indicators (Rando 1996, p. 153) such as:

- *re-experience of the traumatic event*
- *avoidance of stimuli associated with the traumatic event or numbing of general responsiveness*
- *increased physiological arousal.*

From Rando's perspective, grieving traumatic deaths may involve reviewing the trauma as part of grieving. Family members may require skilled resources to assist them to cope. Unless nurses or midwives are qualified and skilled in such work, they should discuss with the family member the option of referral to a counsellor or therapist skilled in trauma work.

Suicidal thoughts and actions

At some point following the death of a child, some parents, and other family members, may have suicidal thoughts. The important distinction, which Hindmarch (2000, p. 133) noted, is that such thoughts or statements are often '*concerned with ending one's misery rather than one's life*'. This is reflected in comments such as:

'*Life is black, there is no purpose*'
'*I can't see the point of going on*'
'*I just want to stop the pain*'

When people make such comments, it is important that health professionals acknowledge and clarify their meaning. Hindmarch provided a valuable description of this process (2000, pp. 132–134) and the following is a summary.

Acknowledgement can be by asking a question such as 'Does that mean you don't want to continue living?' Many people will reply 'No, I just hate feeling awful'.

For those who reply 'Yes', another question can clarify the meaning, 'Do you mean you want to end your life?' Most people will indicate that they think about it but would not act on that thought because of a range of reasons such as having other children to care for. For those people who reply 'Yes' a further question such as 'What would you do?' can clarify degree of intent. A reply might indicate a plan of action combined with reservations 'I think about jumping off the bridge, but I am not sure I have the courage'. A very few people will describe a proposed method with a statement of intent.

At all points during such a conversation, it is important to acknowledge the enormity of pain and distress experienced by the individual. Where the answers indicate intent to suicide, then the health professional needs to explain that they wish to seek the assistance of other health professionals. Because this requires sharing information, it may be important to remind the person that this was part of the original contract of care established at the beginning of visiting. As we noted above, some nurses or midwives feel concerned about their level of expertise to support family members with suicidal thoughts but not intent. If this is the case, then it is important that they work with the family members to secure additional support; for themselves and the family member. This is about accountability for practice and seeking mentoring in unfamiliar roles and responsibilities.

References

Hindmarch C 2000 On the death of a child, 2nd edn. Radcliffe Medical Press, Oxford

Lord JH 1996 America's number one killer: vehicular crashes. In: Doka K (ed) Living with grief after sudden loss. Taylor & Francis, Philadelphia, PA, p 25–41

Rando T 1992 The increasing prevalence of complicated mourning: the onslaught is just beginning. OMEGA, Journal of Death and Dying 26: 43–49

Rando T 1993 Treatment of complicated mourning. Research Press, Champaign, IL

Rando T 1996 Complications in mourning traumatic death. In: Doka K (ed) Living with grief after sudden loss. Taylor & Francis, Philadelphia, PA, p 139–159

13 Setting up a support group for professionals

Before setting up a group the following questions should be considered.

- Is there sufficient interest to start a group? A group of more than 10–12 is generally unwieldy and less than four or five participants can leave members feeling that they have to contribute continually to the discussion.
- Have the main aims of the group been considered?
- Does the group seek to provide support? Does it hope to initiate change in practice where appropriate?
- Are there any theoretical perspectives or models informing the process of the group?
- Who will attend? Will the group be multidisciplinary or of one discipline, e.g. nurses?
- Is attendance a compulsory requirement of employment?
- Will the group be 'closed' or 'open'. Closed means that a set number of people meet regularly and have the opportunity of getting to know each other; this enables trusting relationships to be built. An open group allows for anyone to come and go and is less likely to create close and trusting relationships.
- Are members required to make a contribution or can they attend and choose what they share?
- What will be the ground rules, including a statement on confidentiality?
- How often will the group meet?
- Where is the best place to meet? Somewhere private and quiet, away from telephones is preferable.
- At what time will the group meet and for how long?
- How long will the group run? Is it permanent or for a limited time period?
- Will there be a facilitator? If yes, will it be someone from within the work area or outside? Ideally, a group leader should be someone who has knowledge of bereavement and skills in running groups.

Index

Note: numbers in bold refer to figures, tables and boxes.